Power Eating

POWER EATING

how to play hard and eat smart
for the time of your life

Frances G. Berkoff RD
Barbara J. Lauer
Yves Talbot MD

KEY PORTER BOOKS

Frances Berkoff: To my mother and father, Jean and Bob Berkoff, whose silent applause I hear.

Barbara Lauer: To my family, and my best friend and partner, Denton Hoffman, whose unfailing support has made this so joyful an endeavor.

Yves Talbot: To Lois, Martin and Adam, the greatest supporters of my well-being.

Canadian Cataloguing in Publication Data

Berkoff, Frances G.
Power Eating : how to play hard and eat smart for the time of your life

Updated ed.
ISBN 1-55263-111-7

1 Athletes – Nutrition. 2. Cookery. I. Lauer, Barbara J. II. Talbot, Yves. III. Title.

TX361.A8B47 2000   613.2'024'796
C99-933067-5

THE CANADA COUNCIL | LE CONSEIL DES ARTS
FOR THE ARTS | DU CANADA
SINCE 1957 | DEPUIS 1957

The publisher gratefully acknowledges the support of the Canada Council for the Arts and the Ontario Arts Council for its publishing program.
  We acknowledge the financial support of the Government of Canada through the Book Publishing Industry Development Program (BPIDP) for our publishing activities.

Key Porter Books Limited
70 The Esplanade
Toronto, Ontario
Canada M5E 1R2

www.keyporter.com

Design: Counterpunch / Peter Ross

Distributed in the United States by Firefly Books

Printed and bound in Canada

00 01 02 03 04 6 5 4 3 2

Acknowledgments

This book is a labor of love, based on support from friends and family ten years ago, as well as current friends who have helped keep this book vital.

From the original crew, we thank Patsy Jamieson, Monda Rosenberg, Shirley Ann Holmes, Lance Connery, Donna Hennyey, Pat Latner, Dr. Ron Taylor, Mary Rickett, Ingrid Van Musschenbroek, Barbara Dean, Sonia Baistrocchi and Eric Miller, who named this book!

For the mouth-watering new recipes, our thanks to Joanne Leese, as well as Pat Micks for the research that updates this latest edition. Most of all, we thank Susan Renouf, of Key Porter, for her faith and vision in supporting *Power Eating* and its authors.

An Introduction to a Power Lifestyle

While the purpose of this book is to encourage fitness and power eating, pause first to read the text, don't simply skip to the recipes (the good stuff, as it were). Before you begin eating for performance, you must understand how your body uses the fuel to energize "the machine."

No magic formulas here, rather, good sound guidelines for better living, not to mention beating your opponent on the squash court. The first chapter takes you through the physiology of sport. From chapter two on, we give you a short course in the basics of nutrition, clear up myths and misconceptions and share with you the wisdom of the sports sages on power eating. Our final chapters (just before the recipes) offer an overview of eight sports and what you can expect from them in the way of injuries and fitness benefits. In addition, we give you stretching exercises and menus for training for each of these activities. Power eating for power play.

Eating well, not to mention eating for performance, doesn't have to be tricky, expensive or time-consuming. With leisure time a precious commodity, we have developed recipes that are fast food without being fat food. We've also made them guilt-free eating – healthy recipes using grains, brassicas and fiber without losing any of the robust or tantalizing flavors. Diet is an issue beyond fitness, since there is a growing body of evidence linking what you eat to lowering risks of cancer, cardio-vascular disease and other major health problems.

Power Eating marries your two favorites: health clubs and fast foods. We educate you on the merits of exercise and help you choose the right sport for you. And we offer you food that is high octane fuel without being boring or tedious in the process. We have updated some classics and brought you new ones to love – food into the 21st century.

Fitness doesn't just apply to tennis or jogging. Being fit means having the capacity to enjoy life to its fullest, having the energy to set new limits for yourself, performing at new levels in all areas of your life – sports, the office, with friends and at home. Use this book to train yourself, to develop a healthy body and a new satisfaction with life.

Get ready to enter the next stage of your life: eating smart and playing harder than you ever thought you could. And loving every minute of it.

Table of Contents

Power Eating

A Winning Performance:
food, our bodies and fitness

Why Fitness?

Our bodies, our minds. Everywhere we look – books, magazines, television, radio and newspapers – we are assailed by "recipes" for fitness. What is fitness and why is it so important? Fitness is the capacity we have to meet our day to day challenges. In its broadest sense it can be defined as being fit for work, and for family life as much as being fit for sports. Each of those areas of life presents us with challenges. Each of those challenges represents a harmonious functioning of our mind and our body. An old Latin saying (*mens sana in corpore sano*), "a healthy mind in a healthy body," offers wisdom and a formula for fitness. The formula focuses on a balance of personal reflection, knowledge, action and support (maintenance). Each of these represents an important element in fitness that will help us to live longer, play better and, in all areas, live more fully.

Getting Started: *identifying strengths and weaknesses*

Reflection lets us identify some of our strengths and weaknesses in the practice of a sport. It begins as a series of questions that we ask ourselves to help analyze personal performance. Do I tire easily? Am I cramping too early? Why is my performance decreasing after 10 miles of jogging? Is this the right sport for me? Am I eating the right food? Why am I in a slump with my squash game? These and many more are the questions that we need first to ask ourselves so as to understand why we may be dissatisfied with our sports proficiency. This is the initial process of reflection that will lead to remedial action. Reflection itself is not enough. We need to understand the functioning of our own bodies to interpret some of those phenomena.

Reflection itself is not enough. We need to understand the functioning of our own bodies to interpret some of those phenomena.

Fitness Knowledge Is Power

Richard was training for a long distance bike ride between Montreal, Quebec and Burlington, Vermont. A week before his trip he found that his legs felt heavy and stiff, but he thought they would loosen up on the tour. Testing himself on a hill, he had to give up the struggle and head home. He rested a day and began to increase his consumption of carbohydrates. He tapered his training for the remainder of the week and easily completed the 200-mile round trip.

It has been said we know more about the functioning of our car than we do about our own bodies. Socrates' ancient maxim "know thyself" must apply if we are to become truly fit and to recognize our limits. What do I know about the ingredients of performance? What do I know about the functioning of my body – how it produces and uses energy? What do I know about food that may help to improve my performance? Often the answer is "very little."

Knowledge is essential. You need to know about the various sources of energy and how your body marshals them to enhance your performance at your chosen sport. This knowledge will provide you with the information critical to making an informed choice and acting upon it. This knowledge will therefore enable you in all areas of your life to play better, work better and extend your limits.

Knowledge: *diet and performance*

How does my body change food into energy? Research in the field of human nutrition and performance has, in recent years, yielded very specific information on this subject. It has been known for a long time that endurance performance could be improved and fatigue delayed when an athlete eats a diet rich in carbohydrates. But, how does this work?

It has been known for a long time that endurance performance could be improved and fatigue delayed when an athlete eats a diet rich in carbohydrates. But, how does this work?

The answer lies in the very efficient way our body synchronizes energy production through two different systems. The aerobic (oxygen-requiring) system functions primarily during long distance (endurance) activities. Because these are carried out at a lesser intensity, the body is able to match its delivery of oxygen to the demanding muscle. The anaerobic system (requiring no oxygen) releases energy for short bursts of very intense activity (a few seconds) such as weight lifting, the high jump, tennis strokes and so forth. Exercise physiologists often refer to these systems as being part of a continuum. Most activities are fuelled by both the aerobic and the anaerobic systems but in varying proportions, determined by the intensity and duration of the activity.

	50	60	70	80	90	100
Cross Country Skiing						
Jogging						
Cycling						
Swimming						
Aerobic Dance						
Power Walking						
Racquet Sports						
Downhill Skiing						
Weight Training						

approximate % aerobic demand if practicing the sport vigorously

Glycogen: *our energy source*

Helen, a distance runner, was running in a marathon and decided to keep to the front of the pack. Pushing harder than her normal training pace, she found the first few miles going well. Then her running style became less fluid and she struggled with her pace. By going to the lead too early, Helen finished two minutes slower than her normal time. Had she paced herself more evenly, she possibly could have run the same time or even faster without the pain.

The use of the anaerobic system by an athlete over a long period of time is dependent upon the glycogen stores in the muscles. Carbohydrates not immediately used can be stored as glycogen in the muscles and liver. As the stores become depleted, athletic performance is reduced and fatigue sets in. This is why most long distance or marathon event participants must pace themselves during the event.

It is ATP (Adenosine Triphosphate), an energy-rich molecule, that is the source of energy to both our systems. However, our aerobic system produces twenty times the amount of ATP than our anaerobic system, making it the more desirable performance system for endurance athletes. ATP provides the energy necessary for muscle contraction or any other chemical reaction in the

As the stores become depleted, athletic performance is reduced and fatigue sets in. This is why most long distance or marathon event participants must pace themselves during the event.

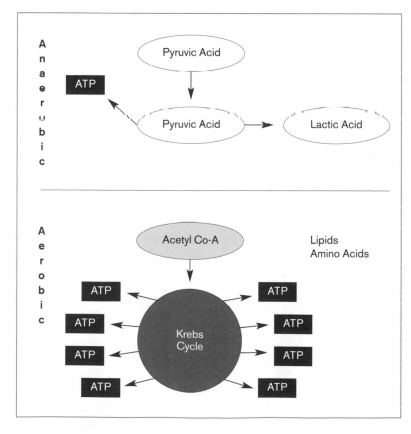

This diagram shows a simplified version of the breakdown of glucose and the release of energy (ATP). The Krebs Cycle is the metabolic process that releases energy in the presence of oxygen. The aerobic system produces 20 times more energy-rich molecules (ATP) than the anaerobic system.

body. ATP is formed from the food we eat, specifically glucose and fat, and is our body's immediate energy source.

The anaerobic system, also called the lactic acid system, is considered a survival system. It functions without oxygen, but produces less ATP (energy units). Lactic acid is a by-product of this system. When this chemical substance accumulates in muscles, the result is fatigue and sometimes cramping and pain. The anaerobic system is considered our survival system because it is the one our body uses to respond to fear, flight or fight. Our body avails itself of this system when short bursts of energy are required (running from danger, lifting a heavy weight). Even during long distance aerobic activities our body will switch to the anaerobic system for a sprint, for example, when cycling, or running up a hill during a marathon.

The aerobic system is highly energy-rich compared to the anaerobic system. It is dependent on the amount of oxygen the body can deliver and make available to the various muscle groups during exercise. No matter how much ATP or energy the human machinery produces, it cannot be utilized 100 percent. Any long distance athlete has to pace himself/herself to conserve aerobic capacity in order to delay fatigue. Upon reaching a steep hill, an athlete's breathing increases in an effort to deliver more oxygen as the need increases. The increased demand can outstrip the supply, that is, the oxygen available to meet the challenge. Then, the body must fall back on the anaerobic system for energy. This produces lactic acid, resulting in increased fatigue and decreased performance.

> Any long distance athlete has to pace himself/herself to conserve aerobic capacity in order to delay fatigue.

The Subtlety of Performance: *VO2 max*

Two friends, Sara and Trudy, trained together regularly and often ran 10 mile races, finishing at about the same time. Recently, they decided to enter a marathon race and trained for the event. During the first 10 miles of the marathon, the two women stayed together. However, halfway through the race, Trudy had to motion Sara to finish ahead of her. Trudy walked to the finish long after Sara had crossed it.

Why are some people better long distance runners? This is explained in part by individual differences in the maximal capacity to use and process oxygen, something called VO2 max. It is believed to be genetically determined.

No one functions at their maximum capacity, so the challenge is to reach as high a percentage of it as possible (% VO2 max). This is called the anaerobic threshold and it can be raised with increased endurance training.

VO2 max is measured in milliliters of oxygen per kilogram of body weight per minute (mL/kg/min). Elite athletes can have a VO2 max as high as 70 mL/kg/min. This means the athlete is capable of delivering 70 mL of oxygen per kilogram of body weight per minute of exercise. Being well trained allows them to exercise at intensity levels as high as 85 percent VO2 max.

VO2 max could be compared to the engine of a car with a four, six or eight cylinder power plant. Genetically, people may have a "four cylinder engine" (i.e. a low VO2 max) and, if untrained, will never increase the VO2 max they do have.

Once the threshold level (the highest percentage of maximal oxygen delivery capacity) is reached, the anaerobic system of energy production is triggered. It is analogous to a reserve fuel system in a car. However, in the human situation, the fuel changes.

The fuel switches over from being predominantly fat (oxygen requiring) and becomes predominantly glycogen (requiring no oxygen). This results in the production of lactic acid as described earlier. A higher threshold level means a person can exercise longer and at a greater intensity before resorting to the anaerobic system.

Fuel as a Factor of Performance

VO2 max is not the sole factor determining performance, of course. As with a car, the quality of the parts, its aerodynamic shape and the octane level of the fuel also contribute to overall performance. Your diet determines the quality of the fuel for muscular work and is therefore of utmost importance.

Two factors determine the type of fuel used during exercise, the intensity of the performance and the duration. These in turn are determined by your fitness level. A combination of fat and glycogen is used during exercise, but the proportion of each, as mentioned before, will vary with exercise intensity and duration.

> Your diet determines the quality of the fuel for muscular work and is therefore of utmost importance.

After 30 to 60 minutes of exercising at moderate (50 to 60 percent VO2 max) intensity, fat supersedes carbohydrate as the predominant source of energy. (Moderate intensity means maintaining a pulse rate of 120 beats per minute for the average person.) Fat in this situation represents an excellent source of energy for the next five to six hours depending on the individual's "aerobic" or fitness capacity.

The athlete's goal in training or performance is to preserve glycogen stores. Exercising too vigorously depletes them far too quickly. Avoiding lactic acid production and the resulting fatigue is the reason to pace yourself during any extended exercise.

Carbohydrate loading prior to long duration exercise and constant maintenance of the carbohydrate supply during marathon running, long distance swimming or any other endurance activity can enhance performance by maximizing initial glycogen stores. It takes at least 30 to 60 minutes of exercise before fatty acids become available as a fuel source.

For most of us who practice sports such as swimming, squash or tennis, the sport period is short enough to leave us relying on our glycogen stores as our main source of fuel. Since we rely less on fat for energy, we need to eat more pasta and grain products and reduce the fat content of our diets.

Finally, another important factor determining our fuel needs is our fitness level. The less fit a person is the more rapidly he or she will move to anaerobic metabolism, therefore increasing lactic acid formation, decreasing the consumption of fat as a fuel and inevitably experiencing fatigue.

Maintaining fitness is crucial for two reasons. First, a lack of training not only decreases the muscles' capacity to store glycogen (i.e., initial glycogen stores will be lower), but in the second place, it forces an earlier (rather than later) switching over to the anaerobic system. A lower fitness status simply means the cardio-respiratory system cannot carry as much oxygen to the muscles nor can the muscles extract oxygen. Training increases our anaerobic threshold for an equal duration of exercise.

Reflection, Knowledge, Action and Support

In order to get started with a healthy mind in a fit body, we have asked ourselves the big questions about our performance and our dissatisfaction with it. We have gathered important knowledge about how our bodies operate: that the aerobic, or ATP-rich system depends on the maximum capacity to utilize oxygen. The anaerobic system, which utilizes glycogen stored in the muscle, is meant for short bursts of energy, often less than a minute. Most sports use a balance of these two systems in proportions dependent on the intensity of the activity, the duration of the energy requirement and thus our fitness level.

Take action by reading about the foods that will fuel you more effectively and improve your performance.

Take action by reading more about the foods that will fuel you more effectively and improve your performance. Use our quick-to-cook, power-packed recipes to get fit and then to maintain your good eating habits.

May the power be with you!

Training to Make Wise Choices

2

A young university graduate who was very active in sports and now sits in front of a computer all day came to Fran for counseling on diet and exercise. Afraid of gaining weight, especially since he was fixing his own meals, he wasn't sure just what he should be eating, let alone how much.

A winning meal plan is simply a matter of balancing your diet. A balanced diet is not just a choice of foods from the four food groups, but balancing all the nutrients needed for top performance. There are more than 50 different nutrients (vitamins and minerals) essential for a healthy body. Too often, we focus on one vitamin or mineral to the exclusion of others, and to the detriment of a balanced diet.

The nutrition recommendations for North Americans encompass eating a balanced diet, reducing the amount of fat in daily diets, increasing the intake of whole grains, fruits and vegetables, maintaining a healthy weight and limiting the intake of salt, alcohol and caffeine. All of this can be achieved through a balanced diet, since within each food group there are a variety of healthy choices. We have to learn to consider the whole universe of food when picking a winning meal plan, and not succumb to the urge to focus our diet on B12 or vitamin E.

We have to learn to consider the whole universe of food when picking a winning meal plan, and not succumb to the urge to focus our diet on B12 or vitamin E.

Beginning with Basics

Since grade school, most of us have grown up with the four food groups (Meat and Alternatives, Milk and Dairy Products, Grain Products, Fruits and Vegetables). These basics of eating are grouped according to their similarity of nutrients, with no one perfect food or perfect food group. In choosing a variety of foods from all four groups, we can expect to meet our nutrient needs and achieve a balanced diet.

Meat and alternatives have fallen a bit out of favor lately. Red meat has taken a beating because of fat, and consumption has dropped. Meat is not the culprit some paint it, if you use lean meat, well trimmed of visible fat. Your body needs two to three servings each day of meat or an alternate such as eggs, lentils or peanut butter. One serving is: 2 to 3 ounces (50 to 100 grams) of lean meat, fish or poultry; 2 eggs; 1 cup (250 mL) cooked dried peas, beans or lentils; 2 tbsp. (30 mL) peanut butter; ⅓ cup (100 g) tofu.

Meat is an invaluable source of protein, iron and B vitamins. In this group variety is important – eating more fish and poultry – while keeping portions smaller. No twelve ounce steaks, please. Half that amount fulfills an adult's needs for one day. Alternates are gaining in popularity as we turn to protein sources such as lentils which are low in fat and high in fiber.

Milk and dairy products provide us with calcium, protein and vitamins A, B2, B6 and D. Once again, adults need two to four servings a day. One serving is: 1 cup (250 mL) milk; ¾ cup (175 mL) yogurt; 1½ ounces (50 grams) cheese. Because of the fat content of some of the dairy group, many people avoid milk and cheese. However, low fat dairy products are an excellent source for all these nutrients since just the fat has been removed. Calcium is extremely important because it helps build bones. Coupled with exercise, calcium is helpful in reducing the risk of osteoporosis, a disease to which women are particularly at risk. Vitamin D, which is found in fluid cow's milk, aids in the absorption of calcium.

Athletes more than anyone know the importance of grain products which deliver B vitamins, fiber, iron and carbohydrates. We need 5 to 12 servings each day of bread or pasta to fuel the eating/performing machine. One serving is: 1 slice bread; ½ to ¾ cup (125 mL to 175 mL) cereal; ½ cup (125 mL) cooked rice, macaroni, pasta. Energy for sport comes from the complex carbohydrates of this group. Until recently, breads and cereals took the rap for "fat." We thought bread and noodles deadly threats to any weight reduction or maintenance diet.

What is a serving of grain products?

1 slice bread
1/2 cup cooked rice, pasta
3/4 cup cooked cereal
1/2 bagel, pita or roll

What is a serving of fruit and vegetables?

1 medium sized fruit or vegetable
1/2 cup cooked fruit or vegetable
1/2 cup juice
1 cup green salad

Now we know the real culprit is what we put on our carbohydrates – the sauces, spreads and fillings that add fat and sometimes little else.

How many of us grew up avoiding leafy greens? Perhaps this explains why we have such a hard time getting the 5 to 10 recommended servings of fruits and vegetables each day. One serving is: 1 average size piece of fruit; ½ cup (125 mL) cooked or raw fruit, vegetable or juice. They too provide carbohydrates, important to athletes, as well as fiber, vitamins A and C, folic acid and important minerals including potassium, iron and calcium.

Of late, various studies have linked different foods from this group to reducing risks of some cancers and heart disease. Fruits and vegetables contain hundreds of phytochemicals – plant chemicals that are essential to good health. These phytochemicals not only make foods attractive and tasty, they provide protection from disease in various ways. Acting as antioxidants, they work to deactivate highly reactive molecules called free radicals. These free radicals have the potential to damage cell structures, making your body more susceptible to cardio-vascular disease and certain cancers. Free radicals also unite with oxygen to form compounds that lead to the build-up of LDL-cholesterol. By deactivating free radicals, antioxidants may help lower disease risk. Some phytochemicals may act to neutralize carcinogens or prevent them from forming, some may influence blood pressure and blood clotting while others may protect the eye against free radical damage, thus preventing or postponing macular degeneration. The research is just starting to discover the numerous other benefits these plant chemicals provide.

This does not mean that any one food is going to work miracles. It does mean you should include plenty of fruits and vegetables (a minimum of five to ten servings a day) in order to get the phytochemicals you need. Mix the brassica or cabbage family (Brussels sprouts, broccoli, cauliflower) with yellow-orange foods (cantaloupe, sweet potatoes and apricots) rich in beta-carotene plus lycopene-rich tomatoes and anthocyanin-rich grapes and blueberries to name a few. It's the balance and variety of all the nutrients that is essential to power, energy and performance.

3 Carbohydrates:
stoking the machine

Bob likes hockey and other team sports, but didn't go out for any team because he couldn't keep up. Although he was tall and big for a nineteen year old, his looks were deceiving. His body was 24 percent fat and he didn't have the strength or stamina to compete. He needed a nutrition and exercise program to lower his body fat level and improve his fitness.

Broadly speaking, the nutrients in food can be subdivided into two categories: the ones that produce energy (calories) and the ones that do not. The energy-producing nutrients are protein, fat and carbohydrates. They give us calories. Vitamins and minerals do not give calories, but they are necessary in order for our bodies to utilize the protein, fat and carbohydrates.

Whether in the act of hitting a tennis ball or schussing down a snowy slope, your body needs fuel for power and performance. Fuel comes from calories – our energy source. Calories are the units of heat produced when our body burns protein, fat and carbohydrates.

Carbohydrate and fat are the major fuels for sport and exercise. Of these, carbohydrate is the most efficient fuel and is burned in its simplest form, glucose. This can be derived from simple sugars (such as glucose, fructose and sucrose) or dietary starch (many glucose molecules linked together in a complex configuration).

Storing Carbohydrates: *glycogen*

When we eat carbohydrates, they are broken down to simple sugars and eventually all are turned into glucose. The speed at which this happens depends on the original form. A teaspoon of sugar will be broken down much more quickly than a piece of bread.

Glucose is the main energy source for our central nervous system, and the preferred energy source for our muscles. After a meal, glucose enters our bloodstream where some remains to maintain normal blood sugar level. This is the body's most readily available source of energy.

> Glucose is the main energy source for our central nervous system, and the preferred energy source for our muscles.

Glucose that is not immediately used is stored in the form of glycogen in the liver and in the muscles for later use. When all our storage places are full, the rest of the glucose is converted to fat and stored.

While glucose is our primary energy source, it has one drawback: it can only be stored in limited amounts. We probably have, at most, 1,800 to 2,000 calories stored as glycogen. Fat can be stored in limitless amounts. With training, however, it is possible to increase the capacity of your muscles to store glycogen. The more you train your body aerobically, the slower you will deplete these stores.

Eating to Prevent Fatigue

It is well known that when muscle glycogen is depleted, fatigue sets in. We recommend your diet be at least 55 percent carbohydrate – more for an elite athlete – for fast and efficient fueling of sport. If you eat 2,500 calories a day, this translates into 1,375 calories in carbohydrates or 344 grams. If you translate this into everyday food terms, 344 grams of carbohydrate could include: 4 cups of milk (one cup of milk has 12 grams of carbohydrate), 7 servings of fruit such as an apple, orange or pear (one serving equals approximately 10 to 15 grams of carbohydrate), 15 servings of bread or grains such as a slice of bread, one-half of a cup of rice or a small baked potato (one serving equals approximately 15 grams of carbohydrate).

Loading up on carbohydrates can also mean loading up on fiber and nutrient-dense foods. Crackers, whole grain breads and cereals are high in carbohydrates, not to be confused with donuts and Danishes which are high in fat.

Since your body can only store 90 minutes' worth of glycogen, it is very important to continually replace muscle glycogen on a daily basis, especially during training. This can be done by eating a high carbohydrate diet regularly, not just on the days you are working out.

Sugar and the Performing Machine

Sugar has been blamed for all sorts of ills and is often avoided by athletes who believe it will hamper their performance. Sugar is not necessarily the villain its detractors tell us. There are several important considerations. Sugar is a concentrated form of energy and simply lacks any other nutrients. This is the reason it is often referred to as an "empty calorie" food. A certain amount of sugar in our diet is not harmful as long as it does not take the place of the essential complex carbohydrate foods.

A certain amount of sugar in our diet is not harmful as long as it does not take the place of the essential complex carbohydrate foods.

The timing of sugar ingestion can affect our athletic performance. It has been shown that having a concentrated form of sugar 30 minutes before exercising can cause a low blood sugar reaction during the sport. However, having a small amount of sugar once the exercise period has started will not result in this problem. Indeed, for many people running a marathon or doing a long distance bicycle ride, drinking a sugared beverage during the event can actually enhance their performance.

Overcoming the Wall Without Carbohydrate Depletion

Carbohydrate loading has long been practiced by endurance athletes as a way to increase their muscle glycogen stores, and thus delay the time to fatigue, or to avoid the all-out exhaustion of "hitting the wall." Formerly, it was believed that if you loaded up on carbohydrates the week before a race, you would maximize the glycogen stored in your muscles.

When carbohydrate loading was first practiced, it was a two-step system: first a depletion bout starting about a week before the event, in which the body's glycogen was used up by exercising to exhaustion for three days and eating a diet low in carbohydrates. This was followed by three days of a very high carbohydrate diet to supersaturate the muscles with glycogen. Although the muscles "soaked up" the glycogen and helped lengthen the time to exhaustion, this method of carbohydrate loading was also accompanied by a variety of side effects including nausea, dizziness, fatigue and irregular heartbeat.

Since exercise is the stimulus for building high muscle glycogen stores, you must be endurance-trained or carbohydrate loading will not work. If you are out of shape, muscles will not store glycogen and instead store fat.

We now advise that people carbohydrate load without depleting. This involves reducing your training somewhat for three to five days before a race, and increasing your carbohydrates to 70 to 80 percent of total calories during this time. This method seems to give the benefits of extra stored glycogen without the unpleasant side effects.

For events that last 90 minutes or less, carbohydrate loading will not help since our normal glycogen stores will last that long. Since exercise is the stimulus for building high muscle glycogen stores, you must be endurance-trained or carbohydrate loading will not work. If you are out of shape, muscles will not store glycogen and instead store fat.

Fat as Performance Fuel 4

Linda, a squash player, came to Fran for counseling on her diet. A busy executive, she had often grabbed high fat fast foods for lunch before her game. However, fat has become a concern since her father died recently of a heart attack. Linda needs to learn the difference between the kinds of fats and how to incorporate more carbohydrates for a high-octane performance.

Fat is our secondary source of fuel, providing the greatest potential energy since our bodies can store it in unlimited amounts. Even for people with the proper amount of body fat in proportion to muscle, approximately 80,000 calories of stored fat are available for conversion to energy. Fat is available as fuel for our muscles in two forms: free fatty acids transported via the blood from fat stores all over our body, and as triglyceride stores within the muscles themselves.

There are limits to using fat as an energy source, primarily because fat requires more oxygen than carbohydrate to burn as a fuel. In order for this to happen, you must reduce the intensity of your exercise. With less intense exercise you have more oxygen or aerobic capacity available for changing fat to energy. It can take at least 20 minutes before fat stores are mobilized for use as energy. However, once fat is being used, you use less glycogen. This is the glycogen-sparing effect of fat which becomes important in endurance events.

Endurance training has a major impact on the increased utilization of fat. First, it results in more free fatty acids being released from fat tissue. Secondly, the capacity of your muscles to burn fat increases, mainly due to the greater activity of the aerobic or oxygen-carrying machinery within the muscles.

If speed is less your concern than increasing fat utilization, make sure your workouts last at least an hour – the longer, the better as long as you keep your intensity low. A too-intensive workout (anything over 70 percent aerobic capacity) will produce lactic acid which suppresses fat mobilization in your body. Your muscles will shift from using fat as an energy source back to glycogen.

When breathing easily meets the oxygen demand, fat is a major fuel source. In general, the higher your aerobic capacity and anaerobic threshold, the greater your ability to use fat.

Your aerobic capacity and anaerobic threshold will affect how easily your body can use fat during endurance exercise. When breathing easily meets the oxygen demand, fat is a major fuel source. In general, the higher your aerobic capacity and anaerobic threshold, the greater your ability to use fat. The physically conditioned or well trained athlete can count on fat for energy at higher exercise intensities, and thus can conserve glycogen stores.

Fat: *the necessary evil*

Each gram of fat contains twice the amount of energy found in equal quantities of carbohydrates and protein. Fats are our source of linoleic acid, an essential fatty acid required by the body. They also are carriers of fat soluble vitamins and provide insulation and a protective enclosure for some of the organs. Butter, margarine, cream, shortening and oils are visible fats. Fats found in milk, eggs, cheese, meats, nuts, avocados and so forth are often referred to as hidden or invisible fats.

North American diets tend to be high in total calories and saturated fat. This means we have a greater risk of developing coronary heart disease, certain cancers and increased blood cholesterol levels. A diet high in fat (where more than 35 percent of your daily caloric intake is from the fats category) also leads to obesity, which is a major concern for many North Americans and is associated with a wide range of health problems.

Health agencies are currently recommending a reduction in daily consumption of fat from all sources, saturated and unsaturated. A high blood cholesterol level is one of the major controllable risk factors for heart disease. In addition to reducing overall fat consumption, it is particularly helpful if the reduction is greater from the saturated sources.

Cholesterol, a waxy, fat-like substance, is a necessary part of all cells of the body. It is produced by the body and is found in animal foods. If excess cholesterol is formed or is not cleared from the blood, it can build up as plaque in the arteries, increasing our risk of heart disease.

Cholesterol travels in tiny droplets called lipoproteins. High density lipoproteins (HDL) and low density lipoproteins (LDL) have been termed the "good cholesterol" (HDL) and the "bad cholesterol" (LDL). It is thought that the HDL carries cholesterol away from the artery walls while the LDL has more affinity for the cell walls, thus increasing the risk of plaque formation.

A high level of HDL and a low level of LDL are desirable. Regular exercise can help raise our HDL levels and a sedentary lifestyle and cigarette smoking can lower them. LDL levels can be lowered by decreasing your intake of saturated and trans fatty acids, increasing your soluble fiber intake and maintaining a healthy weight.

Saturated fats are solid at room temperature and generally come from animal sources — meat, poultry, eggs and dairy. The plant sources of saturated fats are coconut oil, palm oil and palm kernel oil. Saturated fats can raise LDL-cholesterol levels.

Unsaturated fats can help lower LDL-cholesterol levels when they replace saturated fats in your diet. There are two types of unsaturated fats — monounsaturated and polyunsaturated. Although they do help lower cholesterol levels, they still should be eaten in moderation.

Monounsaturated fats are found mainly in olive and canola oils.

There are two kinds of polyunsaturated fat — omega-3 and omega-6 fats. Omega-6 fats are found in foods that come from plant sources and are liquid at room temperature. Food sources include safflower, sunflower and corn oil and some nuts and seeds such as almonds, pecans, brazil nuts, sunflower seeds and sesame seeds. Omega-3 fats are found in fatty fish such as salmon, mackerel, herring and sardines as well as flax and omega-3 eggs. These omega-3 fats help prevent stickiness and clotting of blood. They also help lower triglycerides.

Trans fatty acids are a particular kind of fat created when an unsaturated fat is processed or hydrogenated. Trans fats act similarly to saturated fats by raising LDL-cholesterol levels. These trans fats are found in partially hydrogenated vegetables oils, some margarines, many crackers, cookies and commercially baked products.

It's Your Choice

Reducing fat in our diets can be as simple as making healthy choices. Fat is the most calorically dense nutrient we consume. One gram of fat contains nine calories, versus one gram of carbohydrate which contains four calories. If you make a sandwich of two pieces of bread, a tablespoon of butter and some salmon mixed with mayonnaise, you have a sandwich of about 375 calories. Of that total, 150 of the calories are fat, or approximately 40 percent. If the butter and mayonnaise are cut in half, the percentage of fat is reduced to 25. Cutting back on visible fats and making sensible replacements with other fats is also a virtually painless way of losing weight over the long term. Eating low fat yogurt instead of sour cream, ice milk instead of ice cream, having mustard on a sandwich instead of mayonnaise, and a baked potato instead of french fries can help make the difference in living longer and living well.

Eating low fat yogurt instead of sour cream, ice milk instead of ice cream, having mustard on a sandwich instead of mayonnaise, and a baked potato instead of french fries can help make the difference in living longer and living well.

5 Protein:
building and fixing the machine

John, a body builder, was eating enormous quantities of meat daily in an effort to add muscled bulk to his frame. Although he was eating more than twice the amount of protein his body required, he wasn't building muscle proportionately. Instead, he was gaining body fat and feeling sluggish.

Protein can be used for energy but only minimally since it is not an efficient fuel. Protein is the building block of the body. It repairs the cells that are broken down through the constant wear and tear of our bodies. It replenishes our blood, hair, skin, nails – all our parts.

Protein is also a component of antibodies that fight infection, hormones such as insulin and enzymes that aid in digestion of foods. We get energy from protein, but it is not our body's preferred fuel source. We need protein to build muscle and maintain good muscle tone. Extra protein does not mean extra muscle or strength – only exercise can accomplish that. Extra protein simply ends up as fat if we do not exercise enough.

Many North Americans overeat meat, thereby overeating protein. Extra protein simply ends up as fat if we do not exercise enough.

Protein is made up of nine essential amino acids. These amino acids are essential because our bodies cannot manufacture them and they must be present in the body for protein to be used. We can only get them from food; our body does not produce them.

Meat, fish, chicken, eggs, soy and milk are complete proteins in that they contain all the essential amino acids. Foods such as breads, grains, nuts and seeds are lacking in one or more of the essential amino acids. By combining foods such as nuts and seeds, lentils and legumes you can complete the proteins and meet your dietary needs without eating meat. Food combinations become even more important in a meatless diet in order to ensure that all the amino acids are present to deliver the protein necessary for a healthy body.

For sports such as football and soccer, it is not uncommon for athletes to be asked to gain weight and strength. Increased muscle size, thus strength, is an advantage on the playing field where power and weight score touchdowns. To gain in size and power, an athlete must stimulate muscle growth by exercising against increased resistance; it is not just a matter of eating more protein.

One cup of milk or one ounce of meat, fish, chicken or cheese contains enough additional protein when added to a normal diet to build muscle in the early stage of training. Even as an athlete becomes stronger and needs more protein for the additional exercise performed, another ounce or two of meat would suffice. In North America, most athletes already consume more than enough protein daily to cover the nutritional requirements of extra training.

Vitamins and Performance

6

Dave, A cyclist, went to see his doctor complaining of fatigue. Dave explained that he is spending over $30 a week on vitamin supplements because he doesn't have time to eat properly. He doesn't understand why he is experiencing tiredness and wants the doctor to give him a new vitamin formula.

Protein, carbohydrates and fat cannot execute their functions within the body without vitamins and minerals. If protein and the others are the fuel, it is the vitamins that provide the ignition spark. Vitamins are organic substances and minerals are inorganic. They perform similar functions.

Vitamins and minerals are compounds that facilitate vital biochemical reactions, working alongside protein, fat and carbohydrates. Without them, the other nutrients cannot keep the body healthy. Vitamin comes from the Latin "vita," meaning life. We all require vitamins and minerals to maintain the body's normal metabolic functions.

Vitamins and the Machine

Vitamins can be divided into two main categories: water-soluble and fat-soluble. Water-soluble vitamins, which the body does not store, can be easily destroyed in their food sources by cooking, processing and lengthy storage. This is important to consider when making choices in food preparation. The water-soluble vitamins are the B vitamins and vitamin C. Fat-soluble vitamins are the vitamins A, D, E and K. Vitamins A and D accumulate in the body and can be toxic if taken in excess. Megadoses of vitamin A can lead to fatigue, bone pain, headaches, and changes in your skin and hair.

Athletes and anyone else interested in sports and fitness are concerned about vitamins, and especially with how they might affect performance. Surveys have shown that up to 84 percent of world-class athletes use vitamin supplements, believing that supplements offer benefits both in health and athletic performance. However, if athletes are following a balanced diet, even with the extra energy they expend, supplements are usually not necessary. Extra helpings of broccoli, milk and orange juice contribute more than megadosing with tablets.

If athletes are following a balanced diet, even with the extra energy they expend, supplements are not usually necessary.

Water-Soluble Vitamins: *how they influence performance, health*

Vitamin C aids in the production of collagen, a substance which gives structure to muscles, vascular tissues, bones and cartilage. It helps heal wounds, aids in the absorption of iron and contributes to healthy teeth and gums. Food sources of vitamin C include citrus fruits, potatoes, broccoli, cabbage, strawberries and tomatoes, and peppers.

Since the 1970s, studies have shown that taking vitamin C supplements helps athletes perform no better than if they are receiving the recommended amount from food. The range of tests included mechanical efficiency, strength, distance running, aerobic workup and work capacity. Even so, athletes are often told to ingest massive quantities of vitamin C – amounts clearly beyond those indicated as potentially useful. If an athlete eats a balanced diet with emphasis on fresh fruits and vegetables, it is almost impossible not to receive two or three times the amount of vitamin C needed in a day. In drinking a large glass of orange juice, eating half a cantaloupe, a dish of berries and a serving of broccoli throughout a day, you receive more than three times the daily need of vitamin C. When you look at the full array of vitamins and minerals in foods such as these, athletes should throw away their pills and replace them with fresh fruit and vegetables.

> When you look at the full array of vitamins and minerals in foods such as these, athletes should throw away their pills and replace them with fresh fruit and vegetables.

Vitamin B1 (thiamine) is required to help the body make use of carbohydrates. The more carbohydrate we eat, the more thiamine we need. It is also essential for proper muscle coordination and the maintenance of healthy nerve tissue. Food sources are beef, pork, lamb, poultry, whole grains and enriched cereals.

Because thiamine is involved in energy metabolism, it is often believed that the more we take, the more energy we have. However, studies have shown that any additional thiamine needed is easily acquired through eating a balanced diet. Athletes taking supplements did not perform any better than the athletes eating adequate amounts. Thiamine is contained in so many foods, it is virtually impossible for anyone eating enough calories to meet the demands of their sport not to get the thiamine they need.

Vitamin B2 (riboflavin) helps the body convert protein, fats and carbohydrates into energy. It also helps maintain healthy skin and eyes and build and maintain body tissues. Vitamin B2 is found in milk and milk products, green vegetables and whole grains.

Vitamin B3 (niacin) is essential for protein metabolism, fat synthesis and the conversion of food to energy. Food sources are liver, meat, fish, poultry and enriched grains.

Vitamin B6 (pyridoxine) is necessary for the formation of certain proteins and the use of amino acids by the body. It also helps the nervous system function properly. Pyridoxine is found in liver, nuts, wheat germ, bananas, carrots, peas, beef, lamb and pork.

Vitamin B12 is essential for the manufacture of healthy red blood cells and the synthesis of hemoglobin. Good sources of vitamin B12 include meat, fish, poultry, eggs – all animal foods.

Vitamin B12 supplementation has been somewhat abused in athletics, on the theory that supplementation increases red blood formation and aerobic energy production. Studies of vitamin B12 supplementation, however, found no beneficial effect on athletic performance or aerobic endurance. Vitamin B12 supplements are the appropriate treatment only for a vitamin B12 deficiency; for a well-nourished athlete, they are useless.

> Vitamin B12 supplements are the appropriate treatment only for a vitamin B12 deficiency; for a well-nourished athlete, they are useless.

Folic acid is required for the formation of certain body proteins and genetic material for the cell nucleus. It is important in helping to keep red blood cells healthy. Green leafy vegetables, orange juice, nuts and enriched flour or pasta are excellent sources of folic acid.

Biotin is necessary for synthesizing fatty acids and breaking down protein and carbohydrate molecules. It also helps in the maintenance of the thyroid and adrenal glands, the nervous system, reproductive tract and skin. Sources high in biotin include yeast, liver, kidney, eggs and milk.

Pantothenic acid is essential for the formation of certain nerve-regulating substances and hormones. It is also required for the metabolism of protein, fats and carbohydrates. Food sources are liver, kidney, eggs, peanut products, whole grains and wheat bran.

Fat-Soluble Vitamins: *influencing health and performance*

Joan, a power walker, was afraid of developing osteoporosis and had heard that vitamin D aided in the absorption of calcium. She began to take a vitamin D supplement before each meal to help absorb the milk she was drinking. She arrived at her doctor's office complaining of headaches and nausea.

Vitamin A is important for keeping the skin, eyes and inner linings of the body healthy and resistant to infection. It is also needed for the maintenance and growth of nails, teeth, hair and bones. Vitamin A also helps form the compound rhodopsin (also known as visual purple) which is necessary for good night vision. Beta-carotene, the coloring pigment of many fruits and vegetables, is converted to vitamin A in the body. Researchers are now examining beta-carotene as a factor in reducing risk of certain cancers. Food sources of vitamin A include eggs, milk, liver, kidney, fish, butter and margarine. Beta-carotene can be found in dark green and deep yellow and orange vegetables and fruit.

Vitamin D helps the body absorb and utilize calcium and phosphorus, which are needed to build strong bones and teeth. Good sources of vitamin D are fortified milk, margarine and fish liver oil. A precursor or compound in the skin is converted to vitamin D by sunlight.

Vitamin E helps protect cell membranes and prolong the life of red blood cells in the circulatory system. Vitamin E is found in all body tissues and is important for their proper functioning and health. Nuts, seeds, vegetable oils and leafy green vegetables are excellent sources of vitamin E.

Vitamin E is an important antioxidant. Over the past 40 years, vitamin E supplementation has been advocated for athletes in the hope of improving performance, minimizing exercise-induced muscle damage and maximizing recovery. However, there is currently lack of conclusive evidence that exercise performance or recovery would benefit in any significant way from dietary vitamin E supplementation. Although there appears to be little reason for vitamin E supplementation among athletes, it does not appear that the practice of supplementation is harmful.

Vitamin K is essential for blood clotting. In a healthy body, bacteria in the intestine provide a substantial amount of this vitamin. Food sources are green leafy vegetables, soy beans and liver.

Vitamin Supplements: *do they make a difference ?*

For elite athletes, especially at the world competition level, a very small difference in performance can mean winning a gold or a silver medal. Some coaches and athletes have tried to enhance such performance through vitamin supplementation.

Most research on vitamins and athletic performance has dealt with individual vitamins. Limited research on supplementation with vitamins A and D has shown no effect of either vitamin on performance. Studies with vitamin E did not demonstrate any beneficial effect in a variety of tests. Other work has suggested that vitamin E supplementation might improve performance at high altitudes.

There are very few studies of thiamine and riboflavin supplementation in athletics. Niacin supplementation may have adverse effects through decreasing availability of free fatty acids. There is no research on the effect on athletic performance of supplementation with folic acid.

The general conclusion is that vitamin supplementation has not been shown to improve athletic performance. Chronic multivitamin-mineral supplementation does not enhance physical performance. And a survey of well-nourished men showed supplementation did not affect physical performance.

Some athletes take vitamin injections or pills prior to competition because they believe they can enhance endurance and oxygen delivery in this way. The limited research so far does not lend support to the concept with well-nourished athletes. In fact, taking any vitamin directly before a competition runs contrary to science. Generally, vitamins function as small parts of the greater working whole. This function takes time — not minutes, but hours or even days. Thus, vitamins taken right before an event are still floating in the bloodstream and are useless for improving performance during that competition, even if the athlete was lacking in that particular vitamin. Supplementation may be advisable, however, for athletes on energy restricted diets, but for the nutritionally fit athlete, they have no value.

The best and safest path to good performance is still a balanced diet.

To date, there has been little research on the effects of long term vitamin supplementation and of supplementation with large doses of multivitamin compounds on athletic performance. The best and safest path to good performance is still a balanced diet.

7 Minerals:
inorganic influence on the machine

Alex, an avid softball player, took a salt tablet before heading into the outfield at the start of the league's tournament. It was a hot, sultry day and he wanted to replace the salt he would lose through his exertions. Three innings later, he left the field doubled over with cramps.

Minerals, teamed with vitamins, maintain the body's normal metabolic functions. They are important to body structure and for controlling body processes.

Ironing Out the Fatigue

Iron is the mineral necessary for producing haemoglobin, and haemoglobin is the part of the red blood cell that carries oxygen throughout our bodies. There are two kinds of iron in our food: heme and non-heme. Heme iron is found in red meat and is better absorbed than the non-heme iron found in enriched cereals, some dark green vegetables and certain fruits, such as raisins. It is possible to enhance the absorption of non-heme iron in several ways. Vitamin C is known to enhance iron absorption. For instance, a glass of orange juice drunk with a breakfast of enriched cereal guarantees a better absorption of the non-heme iron. Combining red meat and vegetables increases the iron absorbed from the vegetables. It has also been shown that the tannins in tea interfere with iron absorption. So it is a good idea to save your cup of tea until after you have eaten your meal.

Anemia: *common to the running machine*

Iron-deficiency anemia is one of the most common nutritional deficiencies in North America, identified in many endurance athletes, especially women. When the total haemoglobin concentration drops due to anemia, our muscles do not receive enough oxygen. An anemic person has less endurance and cannot exercise as vigorously because aerobic capacity is reduced.

Iron-deficiency anemia is one of the most common nutritional deficiencies in North America, identified in many endurance athletes, especially women.

We lose iron through blood loss, sweat and exercise. There is the suggestion that mechanical trauma, such as hitting the ground while running, may accelerate the destruction of red blood cells. Runner's anemia is common among endurance athletes, especially female long distance runners. This condition is thought to develop from the destruction of red blood cells due to continual training coupled with low intakes of iron.

Sports anemia is a condition distinct from other anemias. It is characterized by a temporary drop in haemoglobin concentration after a sudden increase in aerobic exercise. The exact cause of this condition is controversial, but it is thought that low iron intakes may contribute to it. Sports anemia appears to be an adaptive, temporary response to endurance training. After a few weeks of training, sports anemia usually disappears.

It is often difficult to correct iron-deficiency anemia without supplementation. Prevention of the problem through an iron-rich diet is the desirable route. If you are not iron deficient, loading up through supplements will not improve your performance. Supplementation, in any case, should only be under a dietitian's or doctor's supervision.

Brittle Bones

Calcium is the most abundant mineral in the body. Our bones and teeth contain most of our calcium, while a small percentage circulates in our blood. This mineral is essential for conduction of nerve impulses, heart function and muscle contractions. Our bones act as the bank for calcium in our body, lending it to the bloodstream if that supply runs low. Our body has a complex system in which hormones interact to keep the calcium level in our blood within a narrow range. This means, that despite locker room stories, cramps in your muscles are not from a lack of calcium.

A great deal of attention has been focused on calcium in our diets of late, because of osteoporosis or brittle bones. Osteoporosis, or loss of bone mass, affects approximately 24 percent of women over 50 years of age. It develops slowly over many years and the key to control is prevention. The person at high risk is typically a postmenopausal, white female of slight build. Contributing lifestyle factors that can further increase risk include high intakes of alcohol, caffeine and protein, smoking and little or no weight-bearing exercise. These act either by reducing calcium absorption into the body, or increasing calcium loss from the body. Osteoporosis is a complex metabolic process that has also been associated with an inadequate intake of calcium throughout the bone building years, which extend into the fourth decade. It is important to note, however, that diet does not stand alone in the prevention of this condition, but certainly is a significant factor.

The most absorbable calcium comes from food, particularly milk and dairy products. Calcium supplements are widely available, but should be used with care.

It is interesting to note that osteoporosis is a disease that affects men as well, although it occurs less frequently in males because of their larger bone mass. Ensuring an adequate calcium intake may also help lower blood pressure, helping to correct a condition that occurs with equal frequency among both men and women.

The most absorbable calcium comes from food, particularly milk and dairy products. Salmon (with the bones), sardines, tofu, calcium-fortified soy beverages, almonds and sunflower seeds are also calcium-rich. Calcium supplements are widely available, but should be used with care. The decision to take a supplement should be made jointly with a physician and a dietitian, after your current dietary intake has been evaluated. We recommend calcium-rich food as the first preventive element against osteoporosis, combined with regular weight-bearing activity, such as walking or jogging.

Sweat of Our Brow

Salt's chemical name is sodium chloride, and it is the sodium part of the compound that concerns us. Sodium is required to maintain a proper fluid balance in the body, and it plays an important role in transmitting nerve impulses.

Sodium is present in our diet in a number of ways. It occurs naturally in a number of foods (dairy products, meat, fish, spinach, beets and celery), is added during processing, and it is added further at the table or in cooking.

Most North Americans consume at least twice as much sodium as they need. This excess links sodium to a number of medical conditions such as high blood pressure. Salt does not cause these diseases, but excess sodium can place unnecessary burdens on your body. While sodium does not cause high blood pressure, it has been identified as one of the risk factors in the development of the disease. This is especially true for those men and women who are "salt sensitive."

There is enough sodium present naturally in our foods to meet our needs. The one time we may need more is during strenuous exercise, especially in hot weather when we may lose significant amounts through sweating. This is easily remedied by lightly salting food before and after exercise. Salt tablets are definitely not recommended. They can be dangerous, as they dehydrate your body by drawing water from body tissues into your stomach to dilute the high level of concentration in the tablets.

Salt tablets are definitely not recommended. They can be dangerous, as they dehydrate your body by drawing water from body tissues into your stomach to dilute the high level of concentration in the tablets.

Minerals That Move Us

Phosphorus is the second most abundant mineral found in the body. A large percentage of it is combined with calcium in our bones and teeth. Phosphorus is part of the high energy compound ATP, as well as DNA and RNA, genetic code materials present in all our body cells. It plays many key roles in energy metabolism, activating other vitamins to function properly and helping our body to absorb calcium. Animal protein is the best source of phosphorus.

Iodine helps regulate the rate at which our body uses energy. It is part of thyroxin, the hormone that regulates our basal metabolic rate. Seafood and iodized salt are the richest food sources of iodine.

Magnesium acts in all the cells of the soft tissues where it forms part of the protein-making machinery, and where it is necessary for the release of energy. It is needed to stimulate muscle and nerve action and also for bone formation. Magnesium is found in whole grain breads and cereals, nuts, legumes, dark green vegetables and milk.

Zinc is an integral part of several enzymes which affect cell growth and repair. It is also important for insulin production, which is essential for regulating glucose in our blood. Food sources of zinc are all animal products: meat, fish and eggs.

Selenium is an essential trace mineral and like beta-carotene, vitamins C and E, is an antioxidant. Selenium is found in fish, cereals, whole grain products, barley and brown rice.

8 Up with Fiber

Becky, a jogger, hadn't included much fiber in her diet before reading all the recent literature on its health benefits. Immediately, she started eating high fiber foods and taking spoonfuls of bran before every meal. Within days she began experiencing gas and bloating, making running impossible.

Most North Americans should double their fiber intake. In the last 25 years, researchers have started to link our Western diet with typically western diseases like hemorrhoids, gallstones and bowel and colon cancers. What makes our modern diet all too different is the lack of fiber. We eat literally tons of processed foods, and the processing takes the fiber out. Finally, we are trying to put it back in.

Dietary fiber is the part of the plant that we do not digest. It goes in one end and out the other. There are many different kinds of fiber which are beneficial in different ways. Fiber can be divided broadly into two categories: the soluble and the insoluble.

Insoluble fibers absorb and hold water. They provide bulk that pushes food through the digestive system quickly. These are the ones that are credited with combating constipation, promoting bowel regularity and treating diverticular disease. The food sources are wheat bran, whole grain breads and cereals, and many fruits and vegetables.

Soluble fibers mix with water in the intestine to form a gel-like substance. This substance acts as a trap that can collect certain waste materials and move them out of the body. Soluble fibers help lower cholesterol and may be helpful in controlling diabetes. The food sources of soluble fiber include oat bran, oatmeal, lentils, legumes, flax, psyllium and pectin-rich fruits such as apples and citrus fruits.

Regaining a Balance

To increase your fiber intake, switch from white to whole wheat bread, use whole grain cereals instead of refined cereals, eat raw fruits and vegetables liberally and consider adding lentils, legumes and flax to your daily diet.

A decided bonus of a high fiber diet is that most foods high in fiber are also healthy for other reasons. They tend to be lower in fat, calories and sodium and rich in vitamins and minerals. And, because they require more chewing and tend to be more filling, these foods are helpful in fighting the battle of the bulge. But remember, easy does it. A high fiber diet started too quickly can make you pretty uncomfortable. So make the changes gradually, drink lots of water and do not focus on just one food. Variety is truly the key to a healthy, high fiber diet.

Fluids: *essential to performance*

9

Adam, a tennis player, was in the midst of a very strenuous match on a hot summer's afternoon. Although he had taken care to drink plenty of water before the match, he was forgetting to replenish fluids during the game. To make matters worse, he wasn't wearing a hat. During the final set, his body seized up and he couldn't finish the game.

Fluids, including water and sports beverages, are more important to performance than any other single nutrient. We can pay too much attention to what we eat and how we train and forget what essentially is the most critical factor to performance: fluids.

Fluids act as our body's cooling system. Whether in a gym or on the road, athletes sweat. Sweating, the loss of fluids through the pores, is the body's way of regulating temperature. Working muscles generate heat and get rid of the excess through sweat. As sweat evaporates, the body cools down. It is a simple and effective way of keeping us healthy, with fluids acting as the key to the mechanism. Dehydration is all too possible as a result of excessive sweating, and moisture loss through breath vapor.

> Fluids, including water and sports beverages, are more important to performance than any other single nutrient.

Heat and Performance

Heat and humidity can impair the functioning of our body's cooling system. Sweat does not evaporate as well or as quickly as in cool, dry temperatures, so excessive heat generated by the muscles can build up. Athletes must take care if they exercise intensively during a heat spell, and must watch their fluid intake very carefully.

Heat, without the humidity, helps sweat evaporate quickly – almost too quickly for you to recognize how much fluid you have lost. Our body's cooling system probably functions at top levels during "dog day" spells, so fluids have to be constantly ingested to prevent dehydration.

Drink Before You Thirst

Throughout any workout during intense heat, you must be aware of how often fluids have to be replaced. Water loss beyond 2 percent loss of body weight impairs your aerobic endurance. For example, if you weighed 150 pounds before your tennis match and weighed 147 after, you have lost 2 percent of your body weight. If this happens, be sure to drink two cups of fluid for every pound of weight loss. Because you cannot count on thirst as a true indicator of dehydration, it is important to drink fluids on a schedule during your workout. The feeling of thirst can come too late for physical well-being.

The physical effects of dehydration include heat cramps, fatigue, deterioration in performance, reduced endurance and heat stroke. These symptoms can hit you any time you lose too much fluid. That is why it is a good idea to weigh yourself before and after exercise, in order to know how much to replenish. Drink before, during and after your exercise, to prevent dehydration.

Contrary to popular belief, cold drinks are absorbed more quickly than warm drinks and do not cause cramping.

Before exercising in hot weather, prepare yourself by drinking two cups of cold water, 10 to 15 minutes before you start. During the course of your exercise, you should drink about one-half cup of fluid every 10 to 15 minutes. After the game, you should weigh yourself and replace any additional fluid loss. One of the best training habits to develop is to drink water regularly, since it can take up to 24 hours for our true thirst to register with our body.

Contrary to popular belief, cold drinks are absorbed more quickly than warm drinks and do not cause cramping. Cold drinks can even give us a headstart with our body's cooling mechanism.

Sports drinks are designed to replace what your body loses during exercise. That's because these beverages contain some sodium, which is lost in sweat, and carbohydrates, which are used by your working muscle. For runners and athletes in training, sports beverages may provide better rehydration than plain water.

Looking for Magic Answers

10

A young wrestler showed up for his annual physical exam concerned about making weight for his school's varsity team. With him was a can of protein powder ordered from a popular wrestling publication which wasn't helping him to make the desired weight in muscle as advertised.

Athletes are always looking for a magical food or drink or vitamin that is going to help them win. These substances are ergogenic aids – substances which are thought to enhance athletic performance. Ergogenic properties have been attributed to a wide variety of nutritional and pseudo-nutritional substances, including bee pollen, amino acids, brewers' yeast, various vitamins, caffeine, alcohol and protein powders.

> In most cases, ergogenic aids are simply more expensive forms of protein, sugars or vitamins.

When the difference between winning and losing can be a split second, it is not surprising that athletes are susceptible to the claims of ergogenic aids. Research to support athletes' stories of the power of these performance enhancers is virtually non-existent. In most cases, ergogenic aids are simply more expensive forms of protein, sugars or vitamins. However, the power of suggestion or superstition can make the difference. When athletes are convinced that certain foods, dietary regimens or supplements can improve their performance, those substances or habits may provide psychological rather than proven physiological benefits. Athletes should be wary of substituting these practices or substances for a sound nutrition program. Serious consequences to the athlete's health and performance can result from such compromises.

Caffeine as a Performance Enhancer

Caffeine is a naturally occurring substance found in coffee, tea, chocolate, cola beverages and some non-prescription drugs. Caffeine is thought to mobilize free fatty acids in the body. The result of this mobilization is the increased use of free fatty acids as fuel, sparing glycogen use and potentially delaying the time to exhaustion in endurance events. Although this may prove to be true for some athletes, it is only valid for endurance events. Caffeine would not be beneficial in short term, high intensity events like sprint running where the body does not rely on fat as a fuel. The negative effects of caffeine should be considered carefully before using it as an ergogenic aid.

Doses of 50 to 200 mg of caffeine (approximately two cups of drip coffee) can change an athlete's perception of fatigue. We may be physically tired, but if we do not perceive the extent of our tiredness due to caffeine ingestion, we may push ourselves to the point of causing injury. That last run down the ski hill is the riskiest one where we can get hurt.

Caffeine as a diuretic promotes the loss of body fluids and can contribute to dehydration. Athletes should not count coffee as a hydration beverage when they are replacing fluids during an event.

Studies have shown that drinking caffeine while eating a high carbohydrate meal just before exercise negates the fat-mobilizing effects of caffeine. It is well known that excesses of caffeine can cause insomnia, anxiety, irritability, stomach upset and headaches. Everyone's tolerance for caffeine differs. It is important to know your own tolerance before an event so you do not put a performance at risk or add a negative to your training routine.

The Phantom of Amino Acid Supplements

There is a common misconception that large amounts of amino acids, the building blocks of protein, are needed to build muscle. Two ergogenic aids jumping on the bandwagon of this myth are protein powders and amino acid supplements. We know our metabolism simply stores excess protein as fat, and excess protein, whether through powders or supplements, can lead to dehydration.

While current research shows that there is an increase in the breakdown of amino acids during physical activity, it is unclear whether all or just a few amino acids respond in this manner. We tend to overeat protein from common sources such as meat, fish and chicken so additional protein or amino acid supplements are unnecessary. Also, taking unbalanced amino acid supplements can interfere with the absorption of essential amino acids.

Alcohol and Its Myths

Alcohol has been used in the past to enhance performance. Studies have shown that it has absolutely no beneficial effect on performance and, in many instances, can cause serious problems at all levels of sports. Alcohol is a diuretic which can lead to dehydration, especially in hot weather. In cold weather, drinking alcohol can contribute to hypothermia.

Alcohol has been used in the past to enhance performance. Studies have shown that it has absolutely no beneficial effect on performance and, in many instances, can cause serious problems at all levels of sports.

Drinking alcohol before an athletic event depresses the nervous system, causing the brain and the muscles to function more slowly and less skillfully. There is nothing wrong with having a drink to celebrate the end of the game, but do not include it as part of the fluids you are replacing. Make sure to drink water first, then the beer or champagne after.

Enhancing Your Performance – No Myths

By far the best way to improve performance is to combine healthy eating with regular training and exercising. If you believe strongly in something, you may benefit from the substance psychologically rather than scientifically. Check with a dietitian/nutritionist or physician before investing money in a new product or changing your diet radically.

Check with a dietitian/nutritionist or physician before investing money in a new product or changing your diet radically.

Common Myths – Conceptions of Sport and Food:

▦ Extra protein is required for building muscle
▦ Red meat is the ideal protein for an athlete
▦ A high fat diet is a healthy way to gain weight quickly
▦ Salt tablets help replace the bodily salt lost through sweat
▦ We can rely on thirst to tell us when we need water

11 Weight Control for Athletes

Donna has been running for years and is a tall, lean, athletic-looking woman. Her weight has stayed the same even as she ate healthily, never restricting calories. After years of running four miles regularly, she increased her distance to 10 miles. Over the course of the summer, she lost 10 pounds. She hadn't increased her caloric intake to support her increased activity.

For many women, the purpose of exercise is weight control or weight loss. A larger percentage of men exercise for fitness. Exercising is a great way to get fit, reduce body fat and, coupled with a healthy, low fat diet, can lead to sensible long term weight loss.

Exercise increases your basal metabolic rate and this effect lasts even after you have completed your workout. The benefit of an increased BMR is the burning of additional calories, which over a period of time can help weight loss. If you exercise while you reduce your caloric intake, you tend to lose more body fat than by just dieting alone.

Dieting to Extremes Cuts Performance

Athletes have to guard against eating poor diets and compromising their performance and health in the effort to lose weight. What you may not realize is that when you begin dieting too quickly the body first loses water and lean muscle mass. The burning up of body fat is a slower process and thus needs to be gradual.

What defines a great body? Obviously, a fit one with the right percentage of body fat.

Another effect of extreme dieting is the lowering of your BMR. Should you try to survive on 800 calories a day and exercise rigorously, your body will try to conserve energy and work more efficiently. This can make weight loss even more difficult.

Society has been telling women for years that they need model thinness to be beautiful, attractive and successful. Such societal pressure can lead to eating disorders that take dieting into the health risk category. What defines a great body? Obviously, a fit one with the right percentage of body fat.

Determining Your Healthy Weight

Great bodies come in all sizes. Healthy weight is the key. A good measuring technique, Body Mass Index (BMI), gives guidelines for a healthy weight. BMI is a formula that compares height in meters with weight in kilograms. The result of the formula indicates whether your size (not just your weight) is in the low, moderate

Body Mass Index

HOW TO FIND YOUR BMI – IT'S EASY

1. Mark an X at your height on line A.
2. Mark an X at your weight on line B.
3. Take a ruler and join the two X's.
4. To find your BMI, extend the line to line C.

Under 20 A BMI under 20 may be associated with health problems for some individuals. It may be a good idea to consult a dietitian and physician for advice.

20–25 This zone is associated with the lowest risk of illness for most people. This is the range you want to stay in.

25–27 A BMI over 25 may be associated with health problems for some people. Caution is suggested if your BMI is in this zone.

Over 27 A BMI over 27 is associated with increased risk of health problems such as heart disease, high blood pressure and diabetes. It may be a good idea to consult a dietitian and physician for advice.

Example: Judy is 5'7" and weighs 152 pounds. Her Body Mass Index is 24.

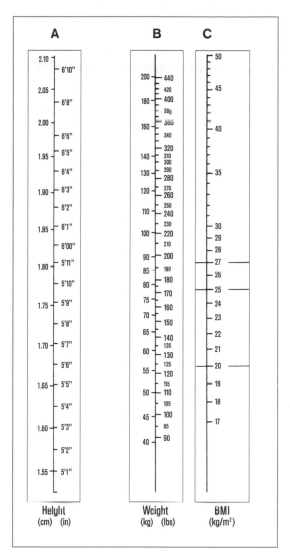

IF YOU FALL BELOW 20 OR ABOVE 27 ON THE BMI RANGE . . .

It's time to reduce your chance of developing health problems. The first and most important thing is to determine why you are not within the healthy weight range and seek the assistance of your physician and dietitian/nutritionist.

Chart reproduced with permission from The Dietitians of Canada.

or high risk zone for developing health problems. Within the "healthy" range of 20 to 25 BMI, there is more than one weight and one clothing size that is acceptable for your height.

The BMI does not apply to an elite athlete. These well-trained individuals have a higher percentage of body muscle, which weighs more than fat. Going strictly by the chart, these athletes might appear to be overweight. It would be more appropriate for them to have their body fat measured. Body fat for elite athletes ranges from 5 to 12 percent in men and 10 to 20 percent in women. Their ideal body composition will vary according to their sport. For the general population, weekend athletes and such, a higher body fat content is acceptable.

Waist to Hip Ratio

Research suggests that it's not just our total body fat but how it's distributed that determines health risks. Specifically, abdominal fat may put you at greater risk for developing heart disease and diabetes. In other words, a pear-shaped body is healthier than an apple-shaped one.

The waist-to-hip ratio can help determine if your weight or shape might cause health problems. To find your ratio, measure your waist and measure your hips around the largest part of your buttocks. Divide the waist measurement by the hip measurement to get your ratio. For men, this number should be 1 or less and for women, it should be 0.8 or less. In other words, your waist should be no larger than your hips.

The combination of waist/hip ratio and body mass index will help determine your weight loss goals.

Every body seems to have a "set" point, a weight at which the body feels comfortable. After dieting, the body will want to return to that weight, often making maintenance a struggle. However, exercise can help change the body's set point, lowering it along with the weight loss.

Diet as a Healthier Lifestyle

Finding your perfect balance of a healthy weight and size is important. Being obsessed with dieting can be harmful to your emotional and physical well-being.

If you are already close to your BMI, then achieving it can be as simple as learning a few new eating habits, or shedding some that have been with you since birth. Finding your BMI, attaining it and keeping it can go a long way toward keeping you healthy and happy in the long term.

For every 3,500 calories that we eat in excess of our need, we will gain approximately one pound of body fat. Translated, that means that if we overeat 100 calories a day for 365 days, we would gain ten pounds in a year. To lose weight effectively, we need to make small adjustments

For every 3,500 calories that we eat in excess of our need, we will gain approximately one pound of body fat.

in our lives, cutting back on our daily intake by 100 calories or so and gently increasing our exercise. These small adjustments become habits we can live with over the long term – not a diet, simply a new way of living.

Increasing exercise begins with frequency, at least three times a week for 20 to 60 minutes continuously at moderate intensity (50 to 80 percent of aerobic capacity, 60 to 90 percent of maximum heart rate). For weight control, your goal should be to expend at least 300 calories per session. In practical terms, this is equivalent to walking three miles or cycling twelve miles. Total energy expenditure is intimately linked to fat loss. By increasing frequency, duration or intensity of your exercise workouts you can proportionately reduce body fat.

Here in North America, where there is plenty of affordable food, over-indulging is too easy. So, focus on eating in a healthy fashion, cutting down on fat and increasing exercise. Make small changes, one at a time, toward improving your performance, your diet and your overall well-being. Today, our goal should be to live longer and to live well.

12 Diet as an Obsession

Beverly was an avid gymnast who loved to eat but needed to stay thin for her sport. She was constantly torn between the desire to eat and a fear of gaining weight. Whenever she gained a few pounds after a couple of days of binge eating, she would fast, abusing both her body and her mind.

There is an increasing incidence of eating disorders among both professional and recreational athletes. Whether prompted by a negative self-image or grueling training, anorexia nervosa and bulimia have life-threatening consequences.

Bulimia and anorexia nervosa are often lumped together in statistics, although they are very different kinds of behavior. Anorexia nervosa is characterized by intense dieting or self-starvation in an unrelenting pursuit of thinness. Bulimia is characterized by recurrent episodes of uncontrollable binge eating (up to 10,000 calories at a sitting) usually followed by purging (self-induced vomiting, laxative abuse, fasting). Experts agree that the incidence of eating disorders, especially bulimia, crosses a wide age range.

Anorexia nervosa and bulimia can have their beginnings in a gym class. It can start as simply as a remark from the coach that a weight loss of a few pounds could lead to increased skill as a gymnast. With females, already at a fairly low weight, this may be accomplished by extreme dieting alone, or in some instances, the extreme dieting may lead to the binge-purge cycle of the bulimic.

Bulimia: *the hidden disease*

Bulimia is a special situation, since it is a hidden disease. Bulimics suffer guilt over their behavior and have low self-esteem. They are often perfectionists and usually excel in academics and/or athletics, but are rarely satisfied with their achievements. These people suffer from a self-imposed social isolation, not just from the secrecy of their disease or preoccupation with food, but from the fear of going out of control around friends or someone they know. Fifty percent of anorexics also are bulimics.

Victims of these eating disorders have their self-image tied to an obsession about their weight. Initially, they may get positive strokes for the weight loss suggested by the coach. This only feeds their already distorted image of themselves. Once entered into the cycle, athletes with anorexia nervosa can reduce themselves literally to skin and bones, losing between 15 to 25 percent of their body weight. In contrast, bulimics usually maintain a near normal body weight. In both anorexia and bulimia, exercise is almost always done alone and for the singular purpose of burning up calories. One study found that 75 percent of anorexics engage in strenuous exercise. Individuals using exercise as a purge may be hard pressed to realize and accept that there is any harm in their behavior. As is the case with dieting, exercise will be praised and seen as a virtue by others.

There is more pressure on some categories of athletes to have a "lean and mean" physique. These include weight-classified sports (wrestling, boxing, judo); the sports that require speed and/or vertical motion – where they are moving their body against gravity (track and field, gymnastics, running); and those where the physique is highly visible (figure skating, gymnastics, dance, diving). These are the athletes that we know are under the most pressure to achieve a low percentage of body fat. If in addition to that, you also have someone who is susceptible to society's pressures of being thin, then you have a prime candidate for an eating disorder.

A Word of Caution to Trainers

If you are a coach, and you suspect some of your athletes of an eating disorder, then you should approach them privately and offer to help them get counseling. They should also be pulled from training since they can injure themselves quite easily. These athletes will deny hunger, pain and injury to keep competing in their quest to be the best. That quest, in an adolescent, can lead to permanent growth damage.

Athletes and fitness participants need to accept that health does not equal thinness or weight loss.

Common observations that may add up to the suspicion of an eating/exercising disorder include: over-exercising with one or more workouts per day; rapid weight loss or fluctuations with the athlete continually dissatisfied with his/her body; a tired facial expression; the same questions, reworded, asked about food frequently; dizziness or fainting; poor muscular development; and a distorted body image.

Athletes and fitness participants need to accept that health does not equal thinness or weight loss. A body needs fuel to run on like any machine. Without glucose, the brain does not function properly. If blood glucose is low when exercising, the muscles feel sluggish and they "starve" the brain in using up all available glucose. This can cause blackouts and dizziness.

A Word to All of Us

If you plan to exercise, eat two hours before to make sure the food is digested. Load up on carbohydrates. And focus on fun, not weight loss. Avoid compulsiveness – every body needs a rest for rejuvenation. Use variety and listen to your body. Do not ignore sensible signals.

There are sports such as wrestling, gymnastics and figure skating, where weight is important and yet the athlete must be strong. If an athlete's body is heavier than is desirable, the weight must be lost correctly, allowing adequate time in order to maintain muscle. When weight is lost too quickly, lean muscle as well as fat is burned for energy and the strength and endurance of an athlete can be reduced.

A scale weight alone should not determine an ideal body weight. The percentage of body fat on an athlete is a better measure and can help the athlete avoid eating too little and exercising too much. Becoming excessively lean will not improve an athlete's performance.

Starvation diets are for losers. They affect athletes in a number of unpleasant ways.

Make sure the weight-loss meals contain smaller portions of nutrient-dense food. Coupled with additional aerobic exercise (30 to 60 minutes), this helps an athlete lose fat and maintain muscle.

Starvation diets are for losers. They affect athletes in a number of unpleasant ways: muscle loss, slower metabolic rate, fatigue, mood swings and loss of strength and endurance. Losing weight through dehydration is even more debilitating, and potentially a killer. Eating properly while losing weight guarantees athletes who will feel like exercising and who will have the energy to do so.

Eating for the Game 13

A football coach we know committed heresy with his team when he switched their favorite pre-game meal of steak to pasta. When the players started grumbling and muttering about losing the game, he quickly asked anyone who was short of energy to sit on the sidelines. No one did, and fortunately for the reputation of complex carbohydrates, the team won the game.

What you eat before the game is as important as when you eat. Timing the pre-game meal can greatly influence the blood sugar level which in turn can make an athlete feel at the peak of condition or slightly off. When to eat is usually determined by trial and error, but meals taken two to four hours before competition seem to give an athlete the edge. This allows the body time to digest the food. If a meal is eaten too close to an event, the digestive system will compete with the exercising muscles for the blood supply, and performance will suffer.

Certain foods such as onions, cabbage and beans which are gas-producing may cause distension of the stomach and discomfort during the performance. Because fats take longer to digest, your pre-game meal should be low in fat and high in carbohydrates. Complex carbohydrates are ideal for maintaining the correct blood sugar level because they are absorbed more slowly than sugar but more quickly than proteins or fats.

> Complex carbohydrates are ideal for maintaining the correct blood sugar level because they are absorbed more slowly than sugar but more quickly than proteins or fats.

Making Your Pre-Game Meal a Winner

The key points for before-game eating are timing (so that food is not left in the stomach) and comfort. Whether you prefer only beverages like water, a blenderized drink or a full meal, successful pre-game eating is a matter of personal choice.

The general guidelines for pre-game meals are:

- Load up on complex carbohydrates (fruits, juices, breads, cereals, pancakes, pasta, rice, potatoes, other vegetables)
- Drink plenty of fluids for proper hydration, avoiding sugar and carbonation
- Stay away from fats and high-fat foods because they delay digestion
- Avoid gas-producing foods (some vegetables and dried beans) and large amounts of roughage (salads, crudités) which can cause discomfort
- Keep portions of protein foods small because they delay digestion as well
- Eat at least two hours before the competition begins

14 Let's Get Physical:
choosing your winning sport

We have profiled eight sports, for both their popularity and for their fitness propensities. Cycling and jogging deliver cardio-vascular tune-ups and conditioning; Nordic and Alpine skiing enhance your enjoyment of winter while toning your body; aerobic dance, racquet sports and swimming offer vigorous aerobic workouts that help with weight control; walking offers fitness without stress; and weight training provides muscle strengthening as well as body toning.

Whether you choose one or mix and match these sports for fitness through cross-training, vigorous exercise will extend your winning performance to all areas of your life. Warming up and stretching are as important to exercising properly as which sport you choose. In Chapter 15 we take you through stretches for all parts of the athlete's body to enhance a winning performance without injury.

If weight loss is your goal in exercising or sport, then make three half-hour aerobic sessions per week your starting goal. And, there is a bonus to regular exercise: it can increase the amount of energy you expend for 24 to 48 hours afterward. The result is continued fat loss between fitness sessions.

Aerobic exercise, as outlined in the sports following, can reduce your risk of heart disease. The benefits of cross-training or exercising through several sports are better overall training, decreased boredom and prevention of exercise "burn out." Besides getting stronger through exercise, your muscles will become more flexible and more resistant to injury. Couple this with good nutrition and you are on the track to living well, living better and living longer.

> Besides getting stronger through exercise, your muscles will become more flexible and more resistant to injury. Couple this with good nutrition and you are on the track to living well, living better and living longer.

If you are over 40, we recommend that you consult your doctor before beginning an aerobic exercise program. This advice holds true even if you are under 40 and have heart disease risk factors (such as high blood pressure). Anyone starting a new exercise program should take it easy during the first few weeks.

To support you in a winning performance, we have developed accompanying training menus. In preparing nutritionally for any sports training, you should have two goals in mind: to train or perform your sport comfortably, and to have enough energy to last the day.

For those of you who prefer to exercise in the morning, whether cycling or power walking to work, have a high carbohydrate breakfast that includes fruit, cereal, skim milk and whole grain bread or muffins. Pack a totable briefcase lunch and snack of nutritional foods such as pasta, fruits and vegetables so your glycogen stores are replenished for the ride or walk home, or for the squash game or aerobic workout after work.

Never let your sport get in the way of maintaining a balanced diet. Don't skip breakfast or lunch because you are short of time. And don't purposely avoid protein-rich foods in order to carbohydrate load. This can lead to long-term performance problems, not to mention threatening your health and well-being.

In general, allow yourself at least half an hour or better after eating, before you begin your exercise. This allows for digestion. Morning or afternoon coffee may give you a "lift," but it is also a diuretic. Large amounts of coffee, tea and colas will cause your body to lose precious fluid and could cause cramping during a workout. Lack of fluid lowers performance, so drink plenty before and after training.

After your workout, refueling is important. Whether this means breakfast, lunch and/or dinner, don't skip meals. Eating a balanced dinner after "pumping iron" or running ensures a proper recovery after any hard effort. Eating enough carbohydrates and drinking plenty of fluid ensures your glycogen stores will be nearly back to normal within 24 hours. Ready, willing and able for another sports session.

With *Power Eating* as your guide, simply pick the activity that appeals to you most, follow the training menus and go for it!

Cycling: *conditioning and weight control*

Cycling is a booming sport. Its popularity and practice has grown to include more than 77 million North Americans. Not only a leisure sport, cycling is the largest single user mode of transportation around the world.

You can expect excellent conditioning and weight control if you bicycle frequently and control the intensity of your exercise. For beginners getting fit, you should cycle three to four times a week, about 20 minutes each time. Cycling while maintaining your pulse rate at 70 percent of your maximum range represents an expenditure of approximately 450 calories/hour. Your maximum heart range is 220 minus your age. This figure times 70 percent will give you your training heart rate, i.e. 220-40 years old x 70% = 126 beats per minute.

Since cycling is an aerobic sport, 70 to 80 percent of your energy requirement during cycling is oxygen. The rest of the time, when you are going up hills or riding short sprints, your system will make the switch to anaerobic.

Cycling utilizes the legs, particularly the quadriceps (thighs), and to a lesser degree the hamstrings, gastrocnemius and soleus (calf muscles). Your upper body is toned because of the constant maintenance of posture.

Many find cycling an aid to sleep and an exceptional activity for reducing stress. For many who are trying to lose weight, cycling is the activity of choice

Training Menus: Cycling

We've prepared menus for pleasure cyclists on a day trip as well as long distance cyclists aiming for a mini-Tour de France. Bon appétit!

A Day on the Backroads:

Totable Lunch
Pasta with Ceci (page 104)
Muffuletta (page 95)
Fresh Fruit
Trail Bars (page 222)
Fruit Juices

Dinner at Home
Grilled Pork Chop
Potato Gratin (page 159)
Spiced Squash Purée (page 154)
Cranapple Streusel Pie (page 233)

"Tour de France Menus"

Breakfast
Yogurt Topped with Truly Healthy Granola (page 75) and
Fresh Fruit
Multi-Grain Toast (page 82) with Jane's Apricot Conserve (page 80)
Fresh Grapefruit Juice

Totable Lunch
Salmon Pâté (page 97) on Rye
French Potato Salad (page 123)
High Energy Oatmeal Cookies (page 222)
Applesauce

High Carbohydrate Dinner
Lentil Salad with Roasted Red Peppers (page 118)
Herbed Spaghetti Squash Parmigiana (page 146) with
Basic Tomato Sauce (page 214)
Green Salad with Light Vinaigrette (page 111)
Multi-Grain Bread (page 82)
Frozen Peach Yogurt (page 220)

since it does not have the same impact as jogging and is less stressful on the various articulations.

Injury Zone:

"Pain in the neck" accurately describes the feeling beginners get when they start and what everyone experiences at the start of the season. It does get better with time and stretching exercises. Neck pains will occur more frequently with the European-style touring handle bars than with the traditional upright ones.

Also a frequent consequence at the beginning of each season, pain in the buttocks can go away. It is often caused by poor positioning of the seat during a long distance tour or a pair of shorts where the seam rubs, increasing friction during the ride. Men seem to ride most comfortably with a seat directly parallel to the ground, while women prefer a seat inclined slightly forward.

Pain in the knees is often a result from poor conditioning or bad adjustment of the seat (either too high or too low). When riding long distances, a certain amount of diffused pain happens and may be related to poor hydration.

Running: *cardio-vascular fitness*

Simple and (relatively) inexpensive, running has become one of the most popular routes to fitness over the past 20 years. Untold millions jog in North America, with hardly a man, woman or child who has not tried this sport, at least once, for recreation.

Its excellence as a cardio-vascular exercise is outstanding when practiced three or more times a week for at least 15 to 20 minutes at an intensity high enough to raise the pulse rate to 70 percent of the maximum heart rate (see cycling). Jogging has other health benefits such as stress reduction, weight loss (for each minute of running, 10 to 15 calories are burned), lower blood pressure and a better cholesterol profile, not to mention a sense of accomplishment.

Running is basically an aerobic sport except for sprinters whose systems switch to anaerobic much more quickly. Speed and efficiency are the result of the positioning of your arms as well as their movements (resistance and coordination of the upper body). Other muscle groups that are called upon during jogging are the quadriceps and gastrocnemius (thigh and calf muscles).

Injury Zone:

Runners are at risk, with 60 percent of them experiencing injuries severe enough to prevent them from training. Knee injuries account for more than one-third of all joggers' injuries. The lower leg accounts for the second greatest number of running

Training Menus: Running

If you are preparing for the challenge of a 10 mile run, whether for fun or in competition, use these high carbohydrate menus for a powerful performance.

Night Before
Lentil and Brown Rice Pilaf (page 160)
Multi-Grain Bread (page 82)
Mixed Greens with Ranch-Style Buttermilk Dressing (page 112)
Moroccan Oranges (page 221)

Breakfast
Fruity Power Shake (page 73)
Multi-Grain Toast (page 82)

Lunch
Soba Noodle Salad (page 114)
Herbed Pita Crackers (page 89)
Nutty Pumpkin Loaf (page 235)
Fresh Apple

Victory Dinner
Blackened Red Snapper (page 207)
Louisiana Rice and Beans (page 172)
Vegetable Packets (page 199)
Lemon "Flapper" Pie (page 234)

injuries. It is wise to consult your physician for any problem (pain) that is a result of running.

Chondromalacia patella (a wear and tear of the cartilage of the undersurface of the knee cap) manifests itself by pain, aching and swelling at the front of the knee. The symptoms are at their worst when weight-bearing or stair-climbing. This condition often results from overuse. Another common knee injury is the pain and stiffness felt on the outside of the knee when running, also called ITBFS (iliotibial band friction syndrome).

Shin splints manifest themselves by pain along the shin when running. Poor track conditions, poor training methods, old or improper shoes and hard surfaces are often the cause. Achilles tendonitis afflicts about one out of five runners and is felt at the lower leg where the calf muscles attach to the heel. Running up and down hills, inflexible soles and certain foot abnormalities can predispose a runner to this injury.

The usual cause of heel pain in a jogger is plantar fasciitis or heel spur syndrome. Typically, the pain is at its worst at the beginning of the run, diminishing before recurring later on, especially the next morning. Poor shoe selection can be a cause. Miscellaneous running injuries include ankle and knee ligament sprains, low back pain, stress fractures, muscle strain and bursitis of various joints.

To minimize the risk of injuries you should: a) wear properly fitted shoes, b) choose a safe route that is soft and c) start slowly. Shoes must fit well, be light and have a flexible sole. Other characteristics of a superior jogging shoe are a resilient heel wedge, reinforced heel cup, molded Achilles tendon pad, flexible mid-sole, padded tongue and studded rubber sole. No tennis shoes, please.

Pick a resilient surface for your jogging – either a synthetic track or a smooth dirt road or grass that is flat and easy to negotiate. Forget concrete or black tar roads. And start easy, with a jog of one to one and one-half miles in 15 minutes or so. You should be jogging for fun and fitness, not training for the Olympics.

Swimming: *toning and cardio-vascular exercise*

This is a singularly refreshing aerobic exercise that can be practiced year round indoors, delivering muscle-strengthening and calorie-burning benefits. One of swimming's advantages over jogging, for example, is the reduced demands on the joints through buoyancy. Being in water lessens the jarring stresses on weight-

---

Training Menus: Swimming

We offer a selection of totable lunches and quick dinners to savor after your body-toning laps.

Lunch
Crudités
Falafel in Pita Pockets with Tahini Sauce (page 171)
Frozen Peach Yogurt (page 220)

Lunch
Mid-Eastern Lentil Soup (page 108)
Herbed Pita Crackers (page 89)
Salad with Herbed Yogurt Dressing (page 112)
Moroccan Oranges (page 221)

Dinner
Penne with Arrabbiata Sauce (page 176)
Mixed Greens with Light Vinaigrette (page 111)
Orange Poached Pears (page 221)
High Energy Oatmeal Cookies (page 222)

Dinner
Grilled Swordfish Steaks (page 209) with
Santa Fe Salsa (page 213)
Grilled Eggplant (page 158)
Lemon Rice Pilaf (page 162)
Seasonal Berries

Dinner
Technicolor Coleslaw (page 129)
Pesto Pizza (page 141)
Fresh Fruit Brûlé (page 232)

Take a break from the rat race and release tension with a midday game of squash. These lunches pack in a briefcase to be savored after the winning set.

Lunch
Gazpacho (page 99)
Lentil Salad with Roasted Red
  Peppers (page 118)
Multi-Grain Bread (page 82)
Oat Squares (page 223)

Lunch
Herbed Pita Crackers (page 89)
Niçoise Pasta Salad (page 115)
2% Milk
Almond Brownie Bites (page 237)
Fresh Pear

Lunch
Pita filled with Middle Eastern Chick
  Pea Salad (page 121)
High Energy Oatmeal Cookies (page
  222)
Fresh Apple

Lunch
Turkey and Patsy's Celery Root
  Remoulade (page 96) sandwich on
  Pumpernickel Bread
Carrot and Celery Sticks
Fresh Grapes

Lunch
Zucchini Frittata (page 138) in Pita
  Pockets
Allan's Marinated Tomato Salad
  (page 127)
Fresh Peaches

bearing joints and ligaments, making fractures, sprains and strains relatively infrequent. Swimming provides good cardio-vascular exercise and tones various areas of the body.

Similar to jogging or cycling, swimming is an aerobic form of energy (at least 80 percent). Because the large muscles of the upper body and lower body are working at the same time, a great deal of energy is expended. For the average swimmer, each mile in the pool represents approximately 600 calories burned. If you were using the crawl at the speed of one mile per hour, you would burn off about 10 calories per minute where a runner would have to run at five miles per hour for the same expenditure.

For aerobic training, we recommend the crawl and back-stroke. If glide intervals are reduced, you can use the breaststroke for training. As with any sport, swimming needs to be practiced three to five times each week for about half an hour to maintain a fitness level. Initially, you can alternate the crawl and the breast-stroke with the eventual goal of completing your session using only the crawl. Because of the overall nature of swimming as an exercise, the trapezoid (neck), deltoid (shoulder), biceps and tri-ceps (arm), quadriceps (thigh) and low back muscles are used.

Injury Zone:

Swimmer's shoulder (pain in the shoulder during the overhead stroke) is a common result of overuse. Tendonitis of the knees and ankles are more infrequent injuries and can be avoided through proper warming up.

Problems many swimmers face are dry hair and skin and sometimes, a chlorine allergy. Wearing goggles helps with eye sensitivity and an emollient cream with dry skin. Swimmer's ear (an infection of the ear canal) can be prevented by wearing water-tight earplugs. If you are swimming in open waters, take a buddy. Supervision is important.

RACQUET SPORTS: *keeping fit while competing*

Racquet sports such as tennis, squash and racquetball generally provide us with social exercise or sport. If you enjoy exercising with a partner or opponent, rac-quet sports are an excellent means of keeping fit. Benefits include decreasing body fat, increasing physical work capacity and improving flexibility, muscle tone and coordination. These games can also provide a healthy outlet for frustra-tion or an excess of competition (where winning at the office isn't enough).

Racquetball and squash are excellent sports for maintaining your cardio-vas-cular fitness and improving your coordination. Although walls limit the surface (from 20 to 40 feet) the ball travels, the speed of its travel makes these fast and furious sports. For those in the fast lane, racquet sports offer a healthy workout in a relatively short period of time. Practiced year round at any of thousands of North American health clubs, these sports allow players of all ages to compete.

Despite the stop/start nature of racquet sports, in vigorous play the action is virtually continuous, representing a good aerobic exercise. Players can maintain their pulse rate at 60 to 70 percent of the accepted maximum for their age. At such a rate, you would burn approximately 9 to 10 calories per minute. Most racquet sports require a 50-50 balance between the aerobic and anaerobic energy systems. A singles tennis match would meet this requirement, although not doubles.

In any racquet sport it is the thighs, legs and arms that are the key muscle groups.

Injury Zone:

The most common injuries are the varieties of tendonitis associated with overuse. Tennis elbow or extensor tendonitis (epicondylitis) occurs in about one-third of all players. Excessive torque in addition to overuse of the elbow are the major causes. Certain factors predispose players to tennis elbow: daily play, a more mature player and a higher level of tennis skill. Beginners can relax, they are less likely to be afflicted.

In most cases, the pain is located on the lateral epicondyle, brought on by arm and wrist activities and is associated with stiffness. Advanced players and those with a forceful serve can develop pain on the inner surface (medial) of the arm if serving too hard or if tension is too high on the racquet. Treatment is rest, anti-inflammatory drugs, ice, stretching and strengthening exercises. When resuming play afterwards, an elbow brace is recommended. Players are advised not to hold the racquet too tight, avoid top spin on the ball and to keep the tension on their racquet to 50 pounds.

With squash and racquetball, injuries are facial or non-facial. The most frequent non-facial injuries are a result of bumping into a wall, while injuries to the face can be from a misplaced racquet, most often self-inflicted by the player.

The nature and speed of this sport make eye protection essential as it could prevent a very serious injury. Poor technique, fatigue, overly aggressive play, ill-fitting shoes and a dirty or wet court all increase the risk of injury to the players.

Weight Training: *building strength for performance*

Weight training is a term broadly applied to a series of exercises utilizing weights to increase strength, i.e., weight lifting. This act of lifting weights or exercising our muscles against a resistance is gaining popularity and acceptance across North America. Weight lifting builds strength and is often used in training for various sports such as swimming, cycling, jogging and racquet sports. It improves the general tone of your body and with proper coaching, can develop both muscle

Weight trainers need protein and carbohydrate in order to build and strengthen muscles. These dinners guarantee plenty of nutrients for "pumping iron."

Dinner
Flank Steak Teriyaki (page 190)
Almost No-Fat Frites (page 149)
Spinach with Rosemary (page 147)
Orange Poached Pears (page 221)

Dinner
Hot and Sour Soup (page 105)
Beef and Broccoli Stir-Fry
    (page 193)
Steamed Rice
Melon Slices with Fresh Lime
    Juice

Dinner
Lean and Healthy Beef Burgers
    (page 192)
Baked Potato with Creamy
    Horseradish Topping (page 90)
Technicolor Coleslaw (page 129)
Berry Berry Shortcake (page 224)

Dinner
Spring Soup (page 106)
Pork with Tarragon Mustard Sauce
    (page 189)
Apricot Bulgar Pilaf (page 181)
Steamed Broccoli
Lemon "Flapper" Pie (page 234)

Dinner
Tortilla Chips with White Bean
    Hummus (page 88)
Diablo Grilled Chicken (page 199)
Santa Fe Salsa (page 213)
Southwest Black Bean Salad
    (page 122)
Fresh Fruit Brûlé (page 232)

strength and endurance. Exercise such as this slows down muscle weakness. If your goal is simply to maintain strength and to condition yourself for other activities you will not need to weight train as frequently. Muscle toning is a process of breaking down muscle fiber, which needs to heal over time before getting stronger. Because of this, weight training involves alternate days of rest and workout whether your goal is to tone or strengthen.

What is a muscle?

A muscle is an organic structure capable of the contraction that produces the movement of various parts of our bodies. Broken down, it is a group of fibers, often called the red fibers for slow contraction and white fibers for rapid contraction, all bound together by connective tissue. The number of fibers is directly related to the size of the muscle. Muscles of your thigh contain many thousands of fibers while a chest wall muscle (intercostal, between the ribs) contains only a few. The tension exerted by the muscle fibers during the contraction produces movement. It is a signal from our brain that triggers the movement.

For example, if we start running, our central nervous system sends a message to the muscles of our thighs and legs to increase contraction and the rate of contraction. This contraction requires energy. A network of capillaries (muscle or small vessels) carries oxygen, sugar and the fat necessary for contracting the muscles. Weight training has the effect of increasing the size of the muscles (hypertrophy), with a resulting increase in power.

Working with weights can improve the performance of any athlete, whether it is to develop strength or size. Because of this, weight training has become an important adjunct to any serious training program. Between two athletes knowing their technique equally well, the one with the greater strength is more likely to win.

Weight Training as Sport:

Weight training decreases fat deposits and increases your basal metabolic rate. People who are muscular tend to weigh more than other people of the same height because of the reduction of body fat (muscle weighs more than fat). The main drawback to weight training as your only sport is that it has little effect on cardio-vascular fitness and flexibility. However, if you include exercises like the stationary bicycle and treadmill in your training, these will provide the cardio-vascular component.

Weight training is primarily an anaerobic sport since it represents short, brisk, intense energy requirements – often less than 30 seconds. All muscle groups can be involved. Generally, a routine alternates upper and lower extremity exercises and lasts up to an hour with a series of three sets of 8 to 12 repetitions of the same exercise. Beginners can expect to train for three one-hour sessions per week for three months. If you are conditioning for other activities, it is at this point you can taper off to once- or twice-a-week workouts to simply maintain your strength.

Injury Zone:

Even if the work of weight lifting strengthens muscles and decreases the risk of injuries in many sports, you still must be very careful. Working with an instructor or trainer is essential to avoid serious injuries. Lack of a proper warm-up is the most common cause of injury resulting in sprained ligaments. It is not uncommon for people to overestimate their strength and use too heavy a load and pull tendons. For regular weight lifters, tendonitis or the inflammation of a tendon and low back pain are also frequent occurrences.

Problems of overuse result in the various tendonitis whether it be biceps, triceps or rotator. Less frequently will you strain or sprain a muscle group. The pain that is usually felt two to three days after performing a series of exercises is related to soft tissue injury. The best approach to weight training safely is to pay attention to the weight you can tolerate and how often you exercise, and above all, to warm up thoroughly.

Skiing: *balance versus endurance*

Skiing, whether downhill or cross-country, is one of the most popular sports of winter enjoyed by 50 million North Americans. Downhill skiing is a thrill, full of excitement as skiers race down hills and conquer the challenges of moguls. It also tones muscles, from maintaining a slightly crouched position with tensed stomach muscles – something like sit-ups.

However, as exciting as downhill can be, it alone cannot provide fitness. Alpine skiers need to condition through weight training and aerobic dance or power walking to maintain cardio-vascular health and to precondition all year long for the winter ski runs. Downhill skiing requires balance and quick reflexes as well as absorption of impact – specifically from the lower back, abdominal muscles and the quadriceps. Most of the work is done by gravity as the skier schusses down the mountainside. Alpine skiing by itself does not get your heart beating at a sustained rate.

The physical demands of cross-country are quite different. Arms, legs – all muscles work together representing an excellent strengthening, toning and cardio-vascular exercise. Because it is a weight-bearing exercise, cross-country skiing also helps maintain bone mass by working bones and joints. Nordic skiers are more likely to use their aerobic system and to need

Training Menus: Skiing

From wake-up until sundown, these menus sustain you on the slopes. Hearty, high carbohydrate breakfasts are followed by hot rib-sticking soups to be shared out-of-doors. Dinner takes the chill off while replenishing your physical reserves for another day of vigorous schussing.

Cross-country

Breakfast
Oatbran Porridge
Breakfast Pita (page 80)
Fresh Orange Juice

Lunch
Mushroom Barley Soup (page 102)
Multi-Grain Bread (page 82) with
Low Fat Cheese
Fresh Orange
Almond Brownie Bites (page 237)

endurance, while Alpine skiers tap their anaerobic system. Your heart beats faster going downhill because of the excitement, not the work.

A measure of how much energy your body does require is the amount of heat produced. If you are a downhill skier you have to dress much more warmly than if you were going out to cross-country ski, simply because the Alpine exercise does not generate the same amount of heat during the activity.

For fitness, a Nordic skier needs to be outside gliding through the trails over hills and through valleys at least three or four times a week. If this is not possible, you may want to round out your conditioning program with aerobic dance or swimming to strengthen your arms and legs.

Injury Zone:

Preconditioning for either Alpine or Nordic skiing is extremely important. If you are out of shape, you are much more likely to have injuries such as muscle pulls and joint problems. Conditioning – whether through weight training, cycling, swimming or aerobic dance – gives you the stamina you will need on the slopes or out on the trails.

Downhill skiing is dangerous only for the very overweight, the under-conditioned or someone with chronic knee problems. If you have any pain or swelling in any joint, you should consult with your physician before skiing.

For skiing in general, how you dress is critical to your health and well-being. Downhill skiers need the warmest clothing, while Nordic skiers need to dress in light, warm layers of clothing to provide better insulation during the varying intensities of the cross-country exercise. Every skier needs gloves and a hat to prevent frostbite of the extremities.

A large part of the injuries to downhill skiers involves the knees and legs, particularly strains, sprains and fractures. Cross-country skiers are more likely to be susceptible to ankle sprains and tendonitis or strains around the hip area because of the stride. Thumb tendonitis from poling is common with individuals who press down with their poles when cross-country skiing. Beginner Nordics can suffer especially, since they sometimes use the poles to propel themselves, creating an almost constant pressure at the base of the thumb.

Aerobic Dance: *toning, bone-mass build-up, calorie-burning and cardio-vascular fitness*

What began in the late 1960s as a televised exercise program for servicemen's wives has rapidly gained a fitness following of millions. Aerobic dance is the choice of many as a fun alternative to running, swimming or cycling. The original high-impact style involves stretching, jumping and running in place to the pounding beat of Top Ten tunes. Lately, low-impact aerobics have grown popular since there is less risk of injury to the musculorskeletal system with its side-to-side or back-and-forth with arm motions. Whatever the type, aerobic dance gives you four main benefits: cardio-vascular fitness, muscle toning, bone-mass build-up and maintenance and finally, excellent calorie burning.

A typical class begins with 10 to 15 minutes of stretching to warm up your muscles and give them the necessary flexibility. Then, prepare to move to the music and raise your heart rate to its target zone over the next 30 minutes to give your cardio-vascular system a workout. Some classes offer a strengthening session after this: sit-ups, leg lifts and several other resistance-type exercises that help with all over toning, especially the legs, thighs, stomach and hips. The best instructors close with a 10 minute cool-down period of stretching and relaxation.

The availability of workout videos for use in your home means you can easily choose to work out in your living room to stimulate your heart and lungs, increase your stamina, improve muscle tone and decrease your body weight. Whether at home or the gym, aerobic dance must be performed at an intensity great enough to increase your heart rate to 60 to 90 percent of the predicted maximum heart rate reserve for at least 15 to 20 minutes three to five times a week before it will improve your cardio-vascular fitness. Low intensity sessions and programs with frequent and long rest periods may not provide the sustained elevation of heart rate required for aerobic conditioning. A complete sport, your routine should involve the leg, thigh, lower back, abdomen, upper extremities and neck muscles.

Injury Zone:

Although aerobic dance is a relatively safe activity, especially low impact aerobics, orthopedic injuries are not unusual. Almost 40 percent of aerobics students experience an injury that either causes pain or limits activity. Believe it or not, the figure is higher for instructors. Fortunately, the majority of these injuries are minor in nature, rarely requiring medical care.

Training Menus: Aerobic Dance

If your choice of conditioning is low impact aerobics right after work, then these dinners make your program complete. Quick, low in fat and offering a balance of all the necessary nutrients, *Power Eating* says it all.

Dinner
Poached Salmon Fillets with Dilled Cucumber Sauce (page 213)
Steamed Red Potatoes and Zucchini
Grapefruit Alaska (page 225)

Dinner
Bruschetta (page 87)
Rosemary Grilled Chicken (page 198)
Classic Risotto (page 180)
Steamed Asparagus
Blood Oranges

Dinner
Spaghetti with Tuna and Tomato Sauce (page 165)
Great Caesar for Two (page 113)
Fresh Grapes

Dinner
Fettucine with a Trio of Cheeses (page 175)
Greens with Light Vinaigrette (page 111)
Fresh Fruit with Raspberry Coulis (page 218)

Dinner
Creamy Golden Soup (page 107)
Warm Szechuan Chicken Salad (page 124)
Crusty Bread
Blueberry Crisp (page 236)

Quick, tasty and nutrient dense, one of these breakfasts will boost your performance after your race-walk around the block. If an evening per-ambulation is more your style, then "dinner in 20" gives you nutrition in the fast lane.

Breakfast
Orange Juice
Chocolate Banana Smoothie
   (page 74)
Bran Berry Muffin (page 76)

Breakfast
Grapefruit Juice
Muesli (page 83)
Whole Wheat Toast
Apple Butter (page 81)
Hot Chocolate

Breakfast
Multi-Grain Bread (page 82) with
Zesty Cheese Spread (page 73)
Bellini Breakfast Special (page 74)

Dinner
Salmon Steaks au Poivre (page 210)
Herb and Garlic Potato Packets
   (page 209)
Spring Asparagus (page 154)
Rhubarb Crisp (page 236)

Dinner
Cucumber Frappé (page 101)
Spinach Salad with Herbed Yogurt
   Dressing (page 112)
Poached Chicken Breast (page 94)
Wild Rice and Orange Salad
   (page 120)
Fresh Nectarine

Over one-half of aerobic dance injuries involve the legs below the knees such as shin splints, foot pains, plantar fascitis (see running), ankle sprains and stress fractures. Back, hip and knee problems are not uncommon. Participants who exercise more than four sessions per week and are over 35 are most likely to injure themselves. Your chances of injury also increase with strenuous workouts, resumption of exercise after a long layoff, poor technique and inappropriate footwear (bare feet have no place in this sport). Finally, the type of floor you exercise on is important. The surface should be firm yet cushioned for resiliency.

Be sure to choose your instructors carefully since their training can be a contributing factor to your injuries. A good instructor will not allow you or anyone else to join a class after the warm-up period of the aerobic dance session has been completed.

WALKING: *stress relief and fat-loss benefits*

Walking, as opposed to running, where the feet are not always in contact with the ground, remains one of the best and most pleasant forms of exercise. It is a great, low-cost way to cope with stress and it provides fat-loss benefits. Recently, walking has evolved into a power sport, a more active and energetic form of the traditional exercise that can still be practiced (almost) anywhere. Because it claims fewer casualties and is initially less demanding than jogging, it is the sport of choice for people who want to maintain a good cardio-vascular condition.

In lower intensity walking, your body uses fat over time instead of carbohydrates for energy. Striding purposefully (about 100 heartbeats per minute) helps you lose about one pound a week if you walk at that rate for 30 minutes five times a week. Your total fitness level also improves from brisk walking: enhanced cardio-vascular fitness and longevity and strengthened, toned leg muscles.

Walking is mainly an aerobic sport. Walkers need to keep their heart rate at 70 to 85 percent of the maximum for their age. Studies have shown that speed walking at certain speeds not only burns more calories than walking, but more than running as well. (For example, if you ran one hour at the average speed of five miles per hour you would burn approximately 460 calories. The same exercise with speed walking would burn approximately 530 calories.) This is attributed to the more dynamic movement of the arms. The muscles involved in walking are mainly those of the ankles, feet, legs (60 percent) and, to a lesser degree, the upper arms (40 percent).

Injury Zone:

Common to walkers are those injuries experienced by joggers but to a much lesser degree. Watch out for possible strains and sprains of the ankle muscles, some shin splints from either poor shoes or walking on too hard a surface – even if the impact is not nearly as great as jogging. Other hazards are those of the outdoors: pets who may chase you, and climate – the extremes of heat and cold. Just as in any sport, hydration is important to performance without pain and cramping.

15 Stretching:
first things first

The stretching exercises following are only part of the routine to prevent a sports-related injury. Before stretching, you need to warm up those cold muscles. Warming up is essential because it prepares you for exercise by gradually increasing your heart rate and blood flow, raising the temperature of the muscles and improving muscle function. Sudden exertion — such as lifting weights or a strenuous aerobic workout — without a gradual warm-up can lead to abnormal heart and blood flow and changes in blood pressure, which can be dangerous, especially for older exercisers.

Warming up is your choice of one of two techniques. Jogging in place or stationary cycling is a full-body warm-up not necessarily targeted to the specific sport or exercise you are about to engage in. General warm-ups use the large muscle groups and are most effective for raising deep muscle temperature. General warm-ups are a requirement before stretching or working out with weights.

Your other warm-up option is a slightly less vigorous rehearsal of the sport you are about to perform. Cyclists, for instance, can warm up by cycling at a light pace.

Five to ten minutes of warming up is usually enough to raise your body temperature and prepare you for stretching. A light sweat is a good indication you have warmed up enough to safely proceed with stretching and your sport.

Cooling down properly, by slowing down gradually in your exercise or stretching for five to ten minutes, can reduce muscle stiffness and prevent the abrupt drop in blood pressure that can occur when you suddenly stop strenuous exercise. Never — we repeat — never stand stock still after strenuous exercise.

When stretching, you must perform the motion in a slow, continuous fashion without jerking or bouncing your limb. Feel the stretch, not the pain. Don't bounce. If you feel pain, you are stretching too hard and putting yourself at risk. Your goal is to limber up your muscles and improve your flexibility before exercising or joining in a sport.

We have separated our stretching exercises by sport, but any or all of them will benefit your body before its winning performance. Ready, set, stretch!

Cycling

Before You Get on That Bike
Before putting foot to pedal, it is very important to stretch your thigh muscles and lower back. No matter the length of ride, stretching can prevent painful injury.
Quadriceps Stretch: Lying on your left side, flex the knee of your right leg and grab the ankle with your hand. Gradually move your hip forward until a good

stretch is felt on the thigh. Hold for 20 to 30 seconds, repeat with the left leg by lying on your right side.

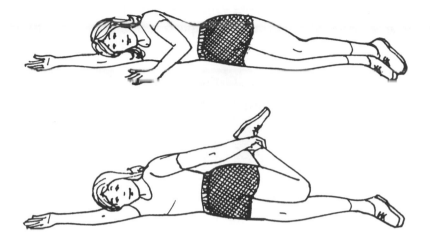

Back Stretch: Lying on your back with arms extended to the sides, bring your knees toward your chin as far as possible without raising your arms off the floor. Hold the position for 20 to 30 seconds then repeat.

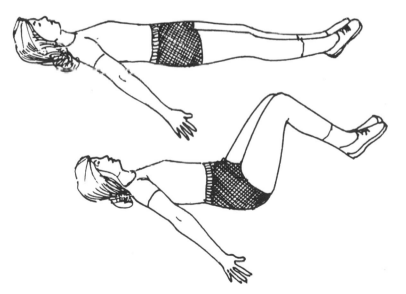

You can also benefit from stretching your gastrocnemius and soleus muscles (calf) and Achilles tendon as well as your neck. (See swimming and jogging for additional stretches.) After cycling, these same exercises can be used to ease tired muscles and prevent stiffness.

Running

Before You Hit That Trail

A 10 minute stretching and warm-up period is just as critical in this sport as in any other in order to avoid pain and injury. Cooling down after your route through the park or laps around the track is equally important and simply a repetition of the quadriceps (see cycling), hamstring and Achilles tendon stretches.

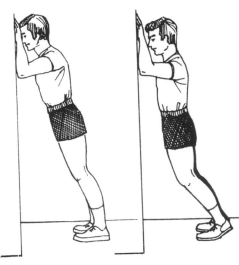

Gastrocnemius, Soleus Muscle and Achilles Tendon Stretch: Stand several feet in front of a wall with your feet seven inches apart and place your outstretched hands on the wall keeping your feet flat on the floor. Gradually move away from the wall by backing up, keeping your feet flat on the floor. Hold every stretch for 30 seconds. Repeat the exercise with your knees bent slightly. Each day try to increase the distance you move from the wall.

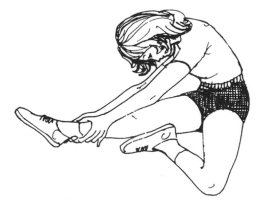

Hurdler Stretch: for your calf muscles and backs of your legs (hamstring). Sitting up, straighten the right leg. Keep the left knee bent, placing the left foot on inside of right leg. Without locking the knees, bend forward at the hip and grab right foot or as far down the leg as you can reach. Pull down until you feel a slight stretch (not pain). Keep the position for 30 seconds and repeat three times. Switch sides, and repeat exercise.

Try bending at the waist, and head and shoulder rolls (see swimming) as other great stretching exercises before you start running.

Power Pancakes (page 79)
Apple Chutney (page 216)

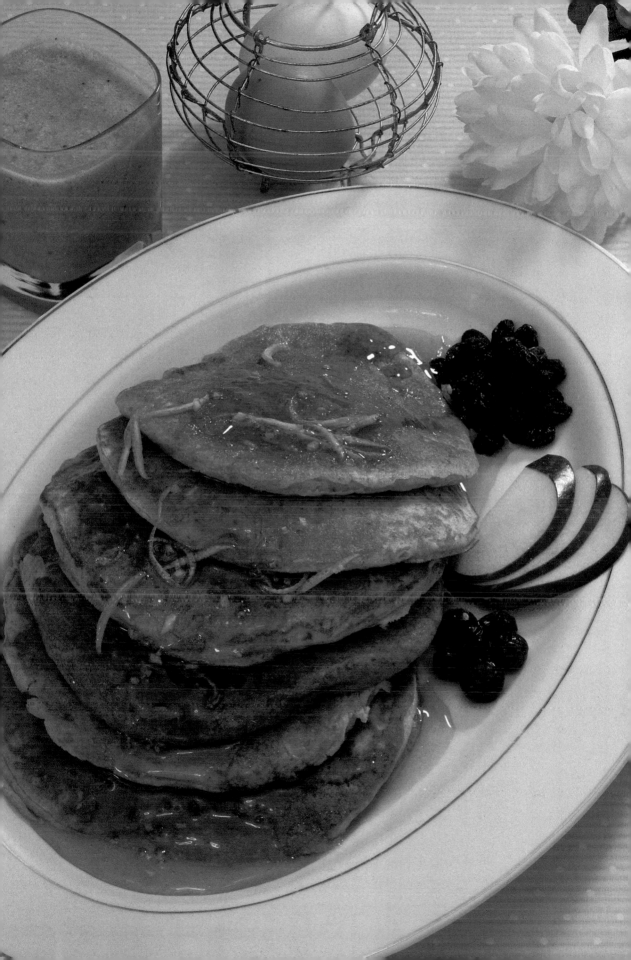

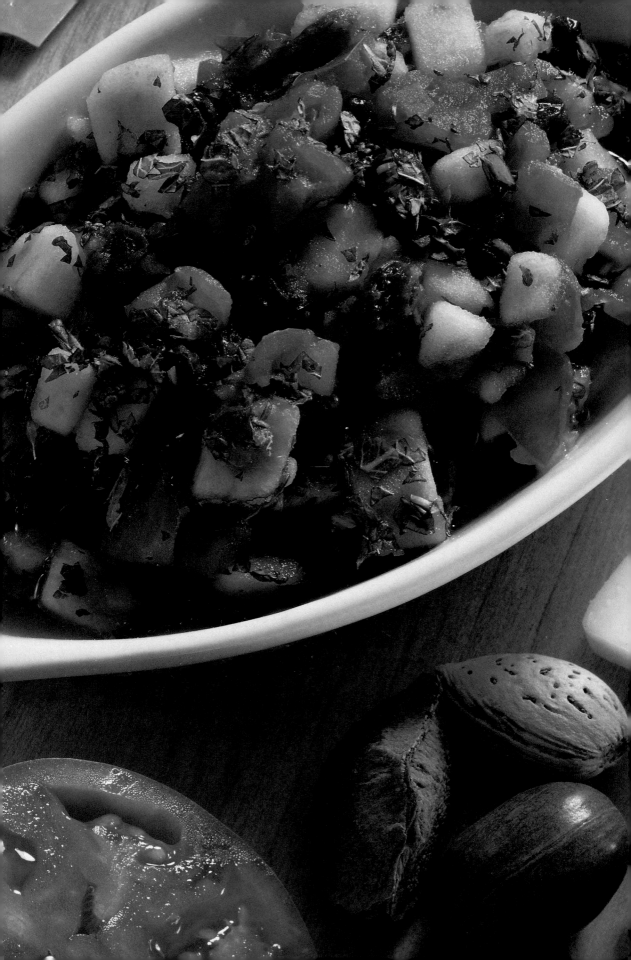

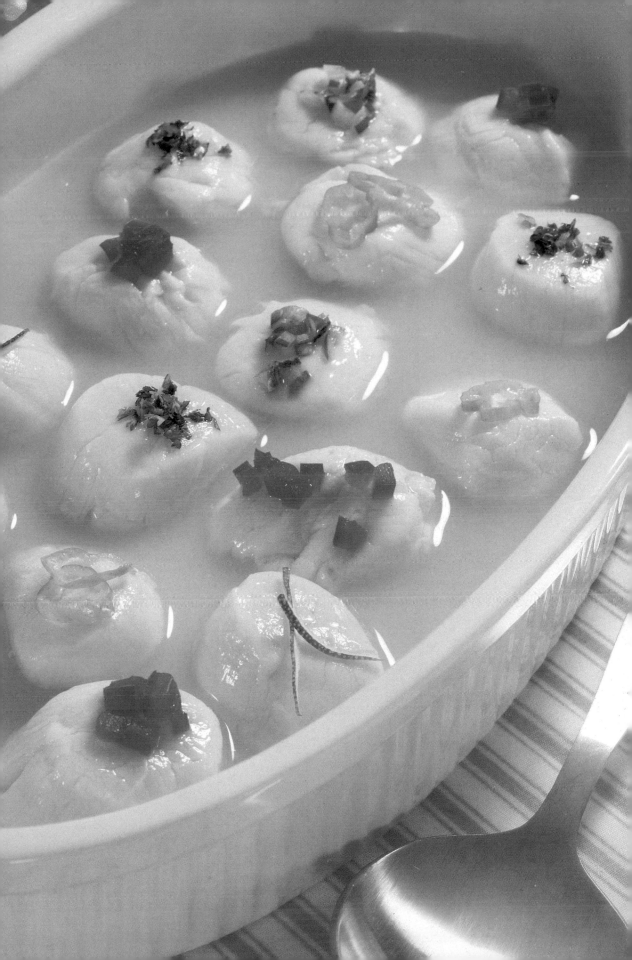

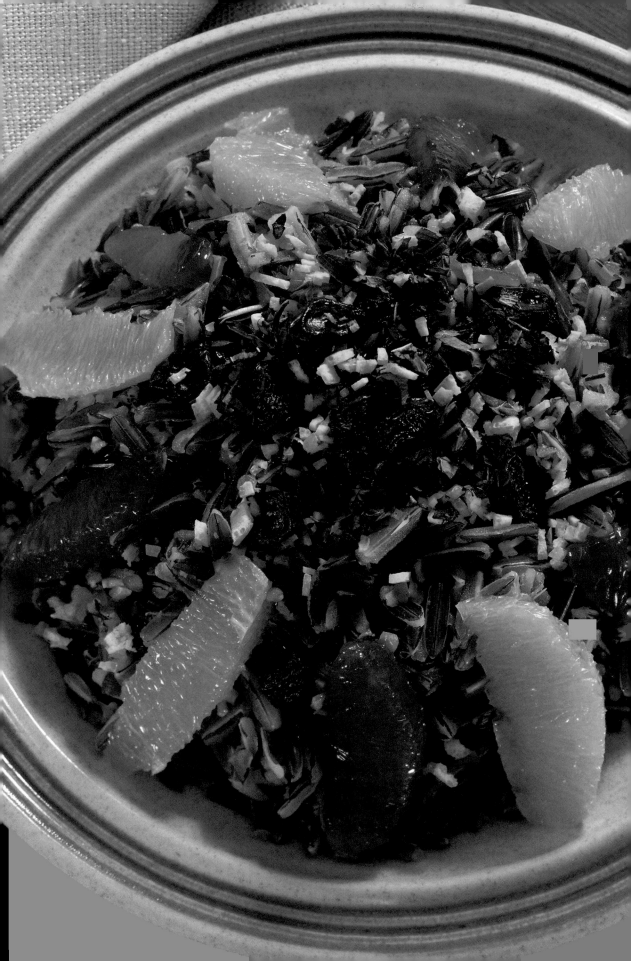

Swimming

Before You Jump in the Pool

Stretching all over guarantees fewer injuries. Begin with head rolls followed by shoulder rolls and biceps and triceps stretches. Finish your warm-up or cool-down period with low back and quadriceps stretches (see cycling).

Head Roll: Keep your shoulders down and breastbone lifted allowing your chin to sink down to your chest. Inhale as you roll your head to the right until your right ear is parallel to your shoulder. Roll your head back, stretching your chin upward. Keep your shoulders down and relaxed. Don't let them shrug up to your head. Exhale, rolling your head towards your left shoulder, feeling the stretch on the opposite side of your neck. Roll your head down until your chin is back on your breastbone. Repeat three times to the right and three times to the left.

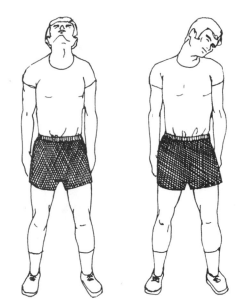

Shoulder Roll: Bring both your shoulders back until you feel the stretch in the front of them. Roll your shoulders to the front until your feel the stretch in the back of them, then roll them back under again to the starting position. Repeat five times.

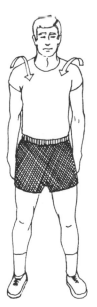

Ceviche (page 91)
Wild Rice and Orange Salad (page 120)

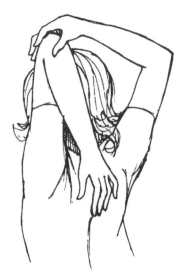

Triceps Stretch: With your arms raised over your head, hold the elbow of one arm with the hand of the other. Gently pull the elbow behind your head, creating a stretch. Hold it for about 20 to 30 seconds. Change arms and repeat this exercise three times on each side.

Racquet Sports

Before You Swing

Stretching your arm muscles, your shoulders and your wrists during warm-up is critical in the prevention of common injuries. Continue with the quadriceps, gastrocnemius, soleus, lower back and Achilles tendon (see cycling, swimming and running) to complete your warm-up before (or cooling down after) an intense game of squash, racquetball or tennis.

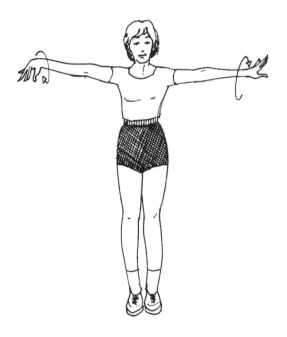

Wrist Stretch: Roll your wrist clockwise and counter clockwise three times each direction, repeating three times.

For more mature adults, a longer warm-up period is critical to preventing the risk of injuries. For people over 40, the warm-up period should last at least 15 minutes.

Weight Training

Before You Lift or Press

At the minimum, you should spend 15 minutes stretching the various upper and lower extremities before weight training (see jogging, cycling and racquet sports for head and shoulder rolls, biceps and triceps stretches, quadriceps and hamstring stretches). The same series of exercises should be repeated to cool down after completing your weight lifting routine.

Skiing

Before You Take Poles in Hand

Warming up for downhill skiing requires exercises that stretch the quadriceps, relax the lower back and strengthen the abdominal muscles. As with any activity, a warm-up period should take at least 10 minutes.

Back Bend: Stand with your thighs and feet close together and breathe deeply, raising your arms overhead. Reach up and back, pushing your hips forward and tightening the buttocks. Hold this position for 10 seconds and then release. If you feel tension in the lower back, come up a bit.

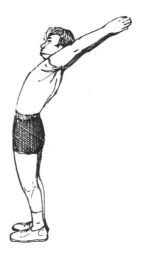

Back Stretch: Lie flat on your back, bringing your knees into a knee-chest position. Hold this position for about 20 to 30 seconds to relax your lower back.

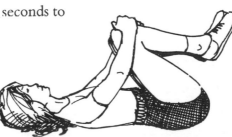

Many cyclists are cross-country skiers in the wintertime since most of the same muscles are used. Not surprisingly, Nordic skiing requires a set of stretching exercises comparable to cycling and running.

Abdominal Stretch: Lying on your back with your knees bent, lift your back (keep your back straight) about 45 degrees until you feel a pull (not pain) in your abdominal muscles. Return to the lying position slowly. Start with 10 per session.

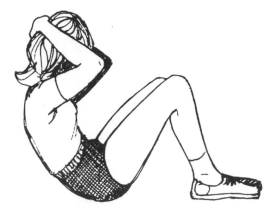

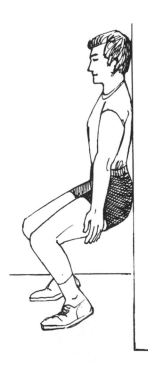

Quadriceps Stretch: With your back against the wall, assume a sitting position (without a chair). Feeling a pull (not pain) in your thighs, try to keep this position for 20 to 30 seconds. Repeat 5 to 10 times, increasing duration.

Aerobic Dance

After the Leotards Are On

Whether at home or choosing a program at a Y or health club, be sure your program has an extended period of stretching before making any demands on the muscles or cardio-vascular system. Follow this series of exercises religiously to prevent injury. A good program will also give you a 10 minute cool-down routine to help you relax after your strenuous workout.

Walking

Before You Take a Stride

A thorough warm-up before your brisk walk should involve the legs, Achilles tendons, hips and lower back (see cycling, jogging and swimming). Stretching before and after you walk will help you avoid many pains and strains.

Hip Stretch: Sit up straight on the floor and bend your knees, placing the soles of your feet together. With your hands, hold your ankles. Gently pull your upper body forward, keeping your back straight. Feeling a pull (not pain) in your groin, hold for 20 to 30 seconds. Repeat three to five times.

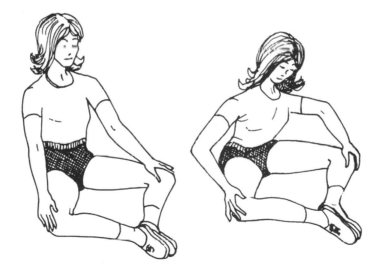

Spiral Twist: Sitting on the floor, cross your right leg over your left leg and bend your right knee. With your left hand grab your right ankle on the right side. Twist your body and place your right hand on the ground, behind you, until you feel a slight stretch (not pain). Hold this position for 20 to 30 seconds. Repeat with the left leg over the right leg.

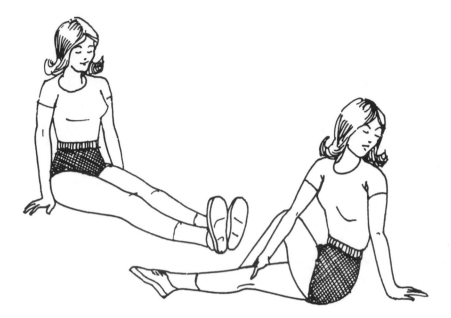

On Your Mark:
athletes to your kitchen

16

Nothing is as intensely welcoming as walking into a home where fragrant aromas and the warm breath of favorite foods kiss your cheek simultaneously with the host. To paraphrase author Gael Greene, we believe great food is like great sports – the more you have the more you want. With this book we offer you food for athletes before events or after. Food to get you fit, keep you active – food for "a healthy mind in a healthy body." Wonderful recipes for the total athlete that are mere child's play in the kitchen, be it ship's galley or country kitchen. Cooking can be as fulfilling a leisure activity as jogging or cycling, and with our recipes it takes less time.

Cooking well (just like living well) takes some upfront organization in the kitchen and pantry, then merely maintenance of critical supplies to manage superb meals when the body is beat. A list of essential cookware and cutlery would include a good set of knives (kept sharp to prevent cutting yourself), a high quality set of non-stick pots and pans (to keep the extra saturated fats out of your life) including a wok and a pot big enough to hold pasta for the whole relay team. There are a few machines we recommend, beginning with the microwave oven. A microwave oven can save eons of time and cut down on dishes and mess in the preparation of some recipes, such as our seafood risotto. So it is an investment in time no busy athlete should ignore. A blender or food processor is a handy gadget that saves time, especially with our power beverages at breakfast time.

For transporting lunches and snacks, have a wide-mouth thermos on hand. Whether it is gazpacho or a hearty minestrone, a thermos keeps it perfect for serving in the office or in the great outdoors. For non-stick cooking and microwaving, invest in plastic and wooden utensils that won't scratch surfaces or cause arcing. Have a set of large (4, 6 and 8 cup) measuring cups in the cupboard for microwaving cereals and other fitness foods without spillage. Heavy duty, durable plastic containers for freezing and glass jars for salad dressings mean extra meals at the touch of a button on those nights you are too tired to cook.

When buying oils, margarines and convenience foods, read the labels. "Lite" may only mean less of something, not fewer calories or less fat. "Caveat emptor" (let the buyer beware) applies just as much in today's supermarkets as it did in the 1500s.

What you should be stocking in your pantry or cupboards, in the way of basic groceries, is a matter of personal taste. However, we provide you with these helpful suggestions, gleaned from the culinary triumphs to come: olive, canola or vegetable oil; white vinegar, red wine or balsamic vinegar; dried pastas: linguine, fusilli, fettuccine, angel hair, spaghetti, buckwheat noodles, orzo, penne; pine nuts; and canned goods: anchovies, sardines, roasted red peppers, lentils, chick peas, white or red kidney beans, tomatoes, tuna, salmon. In the seasoning rack:

salt, peppercorns, cayenne pepper, chili powder, cumin, cinnamon, ginger and nutmeg.

Dried goods should be carefully stored in airtight containers for no longer than three to six months. These include: beans, white long-grain rice, wild rice, Arborio rice and dried mushrooms. All-purpose flours like white flour need to be kept cool, dry and dark in an airtight container for up to one year. Rolled oats and other cereals can be kept on the shelf for up to 12 months as well. Brown rice and dried fruits should only be kept in the cupboard for one month since they can easily go rancid.

The freezer is the treasury of a host of good foodstuffs: bread dough, fresh pastas (ravioli, tortellini, fettuccine), grated Parmesan cheese, pitas, bagels, tortillas, pesto, ice creams and sorbets, bread crumbs, spinach, cranberries, cherries, raspberries, blueberries, homemade soups and stocks. Graham (whole wheat) flour not only attracts bugs, but goes rancid, so is safest in the freezer, along with wheat germ and oat and wheat brans.

What do we keep in our collective fridges to keep us from harm or reward us for a particularly grueling workout? A selection of low fat cheeses, light mayonnaise, several types of mustard, horseradish, dry yeast, a piece of fresh ginger, soy sauce, fresh citrus fruit, parsley and coriander (cilantro), butter, eggs, yogurt, carrots, a brassica or two and skim milk. In the bin on our countertop, you can find garlic, onions and potatoes.

Our philosophy of food and sports is "If it's not fun, why are we doing it?" Obviously, to get and keep in shape. But like exercising, cooking should not be an obsession. According to Mark Twain, part of the secret to success in life is to eat what you like and, we think, to couple this with an exercise you like. Keeping fit is fun, and so is eating healthful food. With the recipes we have designed, eating what you like will be quick, simple and delicious. Success is virtually guaranteed.

To make balancing your diet easier, each recipe shows the values for protein, fat and carbohydrates. When a recipe makes two to three servings, our calculations are based on the larger number of servings. For those of you who are exercising or engaging in sports as a means of reducing unwanted poundage, calories are noted.

Reader, meet good food that is good for you. Fit food to help you live longer, play better and, in general, live well. Recipes geared to a streamlined life that of necessity needs sustenance quicker and better than ever before.

Ready, set, go for it!

★★NOTE★★

All recipes have been tested in a 700 watt microwave oven. If your microwave oven is different, you may have to adjust cooking time slightly.

Breakfast: eye openers

Fruity Power Shake

¾ cup	2% milk	175 mL
1	small banana, peeled and cut up	1
¼ cup	fresh or frozen fruit (blueberries, peaches, strawberries or kiwi)	50 mL
2 tbsp.	2% cottage cheese	25 mL
1 tsp.	granulated sugar	5 mL
2	large ice cubes	2

A good source of calcium, this drink can be whipped up in a hurry before work or working out.

Method
1. In a blender, combine milk, banana, fruit, cottage cheese and sugar.
2. Cover and blend until smooth.
3. Add ice cubes one at a time, blending after each addition.
4. Serve immediately.

Makes 2 servings

1 Serving:
Protein 6 grams
Fat 3 grams
Carbohydrate 23 grams
Calories 143

Zesty Cheese Spread

¼ cup	2% cottage cheese	50 mL
¼ cup	light cream cheese, softened	50 mL
1 tbsp.	chopped walnuts or pecans	15 mL
1 tbsp.	raisins	15 mL
1 tsp.	grated orange rind	5 mL

Ready in the refrigerator, this fruit and nut spread tops any bread and gives you protein and calcium in a lower-fat way.

Method
1. In blender or food processor, purée cottage and cream cheese until smooth.
2. Stir in nuts, raisins and orange rind.
3. Serve immediately or store in refrigerator for up to 2 days.

Makes 1/2 cup (125 mL)

1 Tablespoon:
Protein 1.5 grams
Fat 3 grams
Carbohydrate 1.5 grams
Calories 39

Bellini Breakfast Special

A Fuzzy Navel-type shake that provides most of your morning nutrients for a power start. Complete it by adding whole grain toast or an oat bran muffin.

Makes 2 servings

1 Serving:
Protein 7 grams
Fat 3 grams
Carbohydrate 16 grams
Calories 119

1	medium peach, peeled and sliced (about 1 cup/250 mL)	1
1 cup	2% milk	250 mL
2 tbsp.	orange juice	25 mL
½ cup	2% plain yogurt	125 mL

Method
1. In a blender, combine peach, milk, orange juice and yogurt.
2. Cover and blend until foamy.
3. Serve immediately.

Suggestion
In winter use 1 cup (250 mL) of unsweetened canned or frozen peaches

Chocolate Banana Smoothie

Breakfast in a glass, this chocolate shake is as delicious as an old fashioned fountain milkshake.

Makes 1 serving

1 Serving:
Protein 11 grams
Fat 5 grams
Carbohydrate 42 grams
Calories 257

1 cup	2% milk	250 mL
1½ tsp.	unsweetened cocoa powder	7 mL
1	small banana, peeled and cut up	1
2	ice cubes	2

Method
1. In a blender, combine milk, cocoa powder and banana.
2. Cover and blend until foamy.
3. Add ice cubes one at a time, blending after each addition.
4. Serve immediately.

Workday Menu

Fresh Fruit Juice

Chocolate Banana Smoothie

Bran Berry Muffins (page 76)

Truly Healthy Granola

2 cups	rolled oats	500 mL
1 cup	wheat flakes	250 mL
½ cup	natural wheat bran	125 mL
⅓ cup	skim milk powder	75 mL
⅓ cup	chopped almonds	75 mL
¼ cup	wheat germ	50 mL
¼ cup	flax or sesame seeds	50 mL
2 tsp.	ground cinnamon	10 mL
½ tsp.	ground nutmeg	2 mL
¾ cup	frozen unsweetened apple juice concentrate, thawed and divided	175 mL
1 tsp.	vanilla	5 mL
⅓ cup	raisins	75 mL
¼ cup	dried papaya or apricots, finely chopped	50 mL

Containing no added sugar or oil, this cereal mixture beats any commercial preparation hands down!

Method

1. In a large shallow baking pan, combine oats, wheat flakes, bran, skim milk powder, almonds, wheat germ, flax seeds, cinnamon and nutmeg.
2. In a measuring cup, mix ½ cup (125 mL) of the apple juice concentrate and vanilla.
3. Pour over oat mixture and stir to thoroughly mix.
4. Bake in 275°F (140°C) oven for 45 minutes, stirring every 15 minutes.
5. Meanwhile, mix remaining ¼ cup (50 mL) apple juice concentrate with raisins and dried fruit; set aside while granola bakes.
6. After 45 minutes stir in dried fruit mixture; bake for 15 minutes longer or until golden brown.
7. Let cool completely.
8. Store in tightly covered container for up to 1 month.

Makes 4-1/2 cups (1.1 L)

1/4 Cup Serving:
Protein 4 grams
Fat 3 grams
Carbohydrate 18 grams
Calories 115

Serving Suggestion

Waffles in a Minute: Toast a frozen multigrain or whole wheat waffle according to package directions; top with ⅓ cup (75 mL) mixed fresh fruit. Spoon ¼ cup (50 mL) 2% fruit yogurt over fruit and sprinkle Truly Healthy Granola on top.

Bran Berry Muffins

...portant part of
...festyle. These
...s are winners, with
...n fiber and a fruity taste.

1½ cups	natural wheat bran	375 mL
1 cup	buttermilk or sour milk	250 mL
½ cup	all-purpose flour	125 mL
½ cup	whole wheat flour	125 mL
1 tsp.	baking soda	5 mL
1 tsp.	baking powder	5 mL
½ tsp.	ground cinnamon	2 mL
1	egg	1
½ cup	frozen apple juice concentrate, thawed	125 mL
1 tbsp.	vegetable oil	15 mL
1 tsp.	vanilla	5 mL
1 cup	fresh or frozen unsweetened raspberries or blueberries	250 mL
½ cup	unsalted sunflower seeds (optional)	125 mL

Makes 12 muffins

1 Muffin:
Protein 4 grams
Fat 3 grams
Carbohydrate 19 grams
Calories 119

TIP

To sour milk: add 1 tbsp. (15 mL) lemon juice to 2% milk to give 1 cup (250 mL).
Use an ice cream scoop to divide batter into muffin cups.

Method

1. In a large mixing bowl, combine bran and milk; set aside.
2. In a separate bowl, mix flours, baking soda, baking powder and cinnamon.
3. In a small measure or bowl, combine egg, apple juice concentrate, oil and vanilla; beat with a fork.
4. Stir into bran mixture, add dry ingredients and stir just until moistened.
5. Lightly stir in raspberries and sunflower seeds if using.
6. Spoon into 12 non-stick or paper lined muffin tins.
7. Bake in 375°F (190°C) oven for 18 to 20 minutes or until tops are golden and just firm to the touch.

Spicy Apple Oat Bran Muffins

1½ cups	oat bran	375 mL
½ cup	whole wheat flour	125 mL
¼ cup	brown sugar	50 mL
2 tsp.	baking powder	10 mL
½ tsp.	salt	2 mL
½ tsp.	ground cinnamon	2 mL
½ tsp.	ground nutmeg	2 mL
½ tsp.	ground ginger	2 mL
1 cup	2% milk	250 mL
1	egg, lightly beaten	1
2 tbsp.	vegetable oil	25 mL
1	apple, peeled and diced (about 1 cup/250 mL)	1
⅓ cup	raisins or chopped dates	75 mL

Topping

1 tbsp.	wheat germ	15 mL
1 tsp.	brown sugar	5 mL
½ tsp.	cinnamon	2 mL

Oat bran contains the soluble fiber that helps lower cholesterol. Aromatic while baking, these muffins have a fragrance that will motivate your morning workout.

Method

1. In a small mixing bowl, combine oat bran, flour, sugar, baking powder, salt, cinnamon, nutmeg and ginger.
2. In a large bowl, combine milk, egg and oil; beat together with a fork.
3. Add dry ingredients; stir just until moistened.
4. Stir in apple and raisins.
5. Spoon into 12 non-stick or paper lined muffin tins.

Topping

1. Combine wheat germ, sugar and cinnamon.
2. Sprinkle over muffins.
3. Bake muffins in 400°F (200°C) oven for 18 to 20 minutes or until tops are golden brown and just firm to the touch.

Makes 12 muffins

1 Muffin:
Protein 4 gram
Fat 4 grams
Carbohydrate 22 grams
Calories 140

Wholesome Banana Muffins

Adapted from an old family favorite, this recipe calls for the ripest bananas possible for the very best flavor. Bananas deliver potassium, fiber and folic acid.

1 cup	all-purpose flour	250 mL
½ cup	whole wheat flour	125 mL
1 tsp.	baking soda	5 mL
1 tsp.	ground nutmeg	5 mL
1 tsp.	ground cinnamon	5 mL
½ tsp.	baking powder	2 mL
⅛ tsp.	salt	0.5 mL
½ cup	brown sugar	125 mL
⅓ cup	vegetable oil	75 mL
1	egg, beaten	1
1 cup	mashed bananas (about 2 medium bananas)	250 mL
3 tbsp.	water	50 mL

Makes 12 muffins

1 Muffin:
Protein 3 grams
Fat 6 grams
Carbohydrate 26 grams
Calories 170

Method

1. In a small bowl, combine flours, baking soda, nutmeg, cinnamon, baking powder and salt.
2. In a large bowl, combine sugar and oil; beat until well blended.
3. Add egg, bananas and water; beat well.
4. Add dry ingredients and stir just until moistened.
5. Spoon into 12 non-stick or paper lined muffin tins.
6. Bake in 350°F (180°C) oven for 15 to 20 minutes or until tops are golden brown and just firm to the touch.

Variation

Banana Loaf: Pour batter into 8½ x 4½ inch (1.5 L) non-stick loaf pan. Bake in 350°F (180°C) oven for 45 minutes or until cake tester inserted comes out clean. Remove from pan and cool on rack.

Squash, first played in 1817, comes from the rubbery or "squashy" ball used in contrast to the hard ball used in racquetball.

Power Pancakes

1 cup	2% plain yogurt	250 mL
¾ cup	rolled oats	175 mL
¾ cup	2% milk	175 mL
¾ cup	whole wheat flour	175 mL
¾ cup	all-purpose flour	175 mL
¼ cup	wheat germ	50 mL
2 tbsp.	brown sugar	25 mL
2 tsp.	baking powder	10 mL
1 tsp.	baking soda	5 mL
½ tsp.	salt	2 mL
2	eggs, lightly beaten	2
2 tbsp.	vegetable oil	25 mL

Whether you mix them up the night before or in minutes the morning of, we guarantee you'll find these the tastiest way of getting your complex carbohydrates and fueling a winning performance.

Method

1. In a large bowl, mix yogurt, oats and milk; set aside for 5 minutes.
2. In a medium bowl, combine flours, wheat germ, sugar, baking powder, baking soda and salt.
3. Add eggs and oil to yogurt mixture; mix well.
4. Add flour mixture; stir just to moisten.
5. Heat a non-stick skillet over medium heat.
6. Spoon about ¼ cup (50 mL) batter for each pancake onto skillet.
7. Cook until bubbles appear and underside is golden.
8. Flip and cook other side until lightly browned.
9. Batter can be made ahead and chilled for up to 2 days.

Makes 12 pancakes

1 Pancake:
Protein 6 grams
Fat 4.5 grams
Carbohydrate 19 grams
Calories 140

Note:
1/2 cup (125 mL) fresh blueberries, sliced apple or raisins may be added to the batter before cooking.

Pancake Toppings

Lemon Honey Topping: In a small sauccpan, combine ½ cup (125 mL) corn syrup, 3 tbsp.(50 mL) lemon juice, 1 tbsp. (15 mL) liquid honey and ½ tsp. (2 mL) grated lemon rind; bring to a boil and cook for 2 minutes. This makes a pleasantly tart alternative to other table syrups.

Yogurt Honey Sauce: In a measuring cup, combine 1 cup (500 mL) 2% plain yogurt, 3 tbsp. (50 mL) liquid honey and ½ tsp. (2 mL) cinnamon. Serve with Power Pancakes.

Breakfast Pita

For lovers of scrambled eggs, these are as light and fluffy as traditional but contain half the fat. For a change, substitute Zucchini Frittata (page 138) for the scrambled eggs.

Makes 1 serving

1 Serving:
Protein 18 grams
Fat 7 grams
Carbohydrate 33 grams
Calories 267

1	egg	1
1	egg white	1
1 tbsp.	skim milk or water	15 mL
1 to 2 tbsp.	shredded low-fat mozzarella or cheddar cheese	15 to 25 mL
	salt and pepper	
1	whole wheat pita (about 6 inches/16 cm)	1

Microwave Method

1. In microwaveable bowl, beat egg, egg white and milk with a fork.
2. Microwave at High for about 1 minute or until set but moist, stirring twice.
3. Stir in cheese, add salt and pepper to taste. Let stand for 2 minutes.
4. Meanwhile, wrap pita in paper toweling and microwave at High for 10 seconds or until warm.
5. Cut in half and fill with scrambled eggs.

Jane's Apricot Conserve

A lighter version of the Lauer family favorite, this spread can be made literally in minutes and complements any whole grain toast.

Makes 2-1/4 to 2-1/2 cups (550 to 625 mL)

1 Tablespoon:
Carbohydrate 8 grams
Calories 32

2 cups	dried apricots (about ½ lb/250 g)	500 mL
1	14oz/398 mL can unsweetened, crushed pineapple	1
¼ cup	granulated sugar	50 mL
2 tsp.	lemon juice	10 mL

Microwave Method

1. Using kitchen shears, cut apricots in half and combine with crushed pineapple in bowl of food processor.
2. Coarsely chop with pulsing motion.
3. Transfer to 8 cup (2 L) microwaveable measure or casserole.
4. Cover with vented plastic wrap; microwave at High for 8 minutes, stirring once.
5. Add sugar and lemon juice; microwave at Medium (50%) for 8 minutes, stirring once.
6. Cool and store in refrigerator for up to 1 month.

Apple Butter

½	medium orange	½
2	medium apples, peeled, cored and cut in large chunks	2
1 tbsp.	brown sugar	15 mL
½ tsp.	ground cinnamon	2 mL
¼ tsp.	ground allspice or cloves	1 mL

Method
1. Grate orange rind and squeeze the juice from orange; in a small saucepan combine juice, rind and apple.
2. Add sugar; cover and cook over medium–low heat, stirring occasionally to break up fruit until mixture is very thick, about 25 to 30 minutes.
3. Stir in cinnamon and allspice.
4. Cool and store in refrigerator for up to a week or freeze.

Serving Suggestion
Fruit 'n' Cheese Plate: Serve ⅓ cup (75 mL) cottage cheese topped with 2 tbsp. (25 mL) apple butter in a small custard cup or ramekin. Use the mixture to spread on fruit wedges (e.g., apple, pear, orange, nectarine) and wholemeal bran biscuits.

Lower in sugar than either jams or traditional apple butter, this flavorful spread is great on pancakes, scones and other breakfast treats.

Makes 1/2 cup (125 mL)

1 Tablespoon:
Carbohydrate 7 grams
Calories 28

Multi-Grain Bread

Well worth the effort to make at home, this dense, nutty loaf is superb alone, toasted or as part of a wholesome sandwich. Because of the quick-rise yeast and no-knead method, the time to create this loaf is reduced significantly.

Makes 1 loaf

1 Slice:
Protein 4 grams
Fat 3 grams
Carbohydrate 23 grams
Calories 135

½ cup	multi-grain cereal (e.g., Red River®, 5-grain, 7-grain)	125 mL
1½ cups	boiling water	375 mL
3 tbsp.	honey	50 mL
2 tbsp.	vegetable oil	25 mL
2 cups	all-purpose flour, divided	500 mL
¾ cup	whole wheat flour	175 mL
¼ cup	oat bran or natural wheat bran	50 mL
1	8 g envelope quick-rise yeast	1
1 tsp.	granulated sugar	5 mL
½ tsp.	salt	2 mL
1	egg	1

Method

1. In a small bowl, combine cereal with boiling water and set aside for 10 minutes.
2. Stir in honey and oil; heat until hot (125° to 130°F/ 50° to 55°C).
3. In a large bowl, mix 1 cup (250 mL) of the all-purpose flour, whole wheat flour, bran, yeast, sugar and salt.
4. Beat in hot cereal mixture; add egg.
5. Using electric mixer, beat for 2 minutes at medium speed.
6. Stir in enough of the remaining all-purpose flour to make a stiff batter.
7. With floured hands, pat dough into a 9 x 5 inch (2 L) non-stick loaf pan.
8. Cover with lightly greased plastic wrap.
9. Turn oven to 200°F (100°C) for 2 minutes; turn off.
10. Place bread in oven and let rise until doubled, about 40 to 60 minutes.
11. Remove from oven and remove plastic wrap.
12. Bake at 375°F (190°C) for 35 to 40 minutes or until bottom of loaf sounds hollow when tapped.
13. Remove from pan; cool on wire rack.

Food Processor Method

1. Soak cereal in boiling water as directed in recipe.
2. Insert the blade recommended in food processor manual.
3. In food processor, combine all-purpose flour, whole wheat flour, bran, yeast, sugar and salt; add cereal with water.
4. Mix honey, oil and egg together.
5. With food processor running, add honey mixture.
6. Process until dough forms a ball.
7. If too dry, add 1 tbsp. (15 mL) water; if too sticky, add 1 tbsp. (15 mL) flour.
8. Process for 45 to 60 seconds.
9. Pat into pan, let rise and bake as directed in recipe.

Muesli

½ cup	rolled oats	125 mL
¼ cup	warm 2% milk	50 mL
½ cup	2% plain yogurt	125 mL
2 tbsp.	honey	25 mL
1 tbsp.	lemon juice	15 mL
1	apple, cored and grated or diced	1
1 cup	strawberries, raspberries or blueberries	250 mL
2 tbsp.	chopped toasted almonds or hazelnuts	25 mL

Adapted from Chef Michael Bonacini's recipe, this healthful Swiss favorite was the original "Spa Cuisine."

Method

1. In a small bowl, combine rolled oats and warm milk; allow to soften for 15 minutes.
2. Mix in yogurt, honey and lemon juice.
3. Add apples, berries and nuts.
4. Serve immediately or cover and refrigerate for up to 2 days.

Makes 2 servings

1 Serving:
Protein 8 grams
Fat 6 grams
Carbohydrate 55 grams
Calories 306

Microwaved Breakfast Cereals

For individual servings combine ⅛ tsp. (0.5 mL) salt, cereal and very hot water in a large cereal bowl as indicated below. Stir once during cooking; let stand.

Cereal	Amount	Hot water	Approximate Cooking Time at High	Standing Time
quick oatmeal	¼ cup (50 mL)	½ cup (125 mL)	1½ to 2 min.	1 min.
oat bran	¼ cup (50 mL)	½ cup (125 mL)	1 to 1½ min.	1 min.
regular rolled oats	*¼ cup (50 mL)	½ cup (125 mL)	3 to 4 min.	2 min.
cream of wheat	*2½ tbsp. (30 mL)	1 cup (250 mL)	3 to 4 min.	1 min.
multi-grain cereal (e.g., Red River®, 5-grain or 7-grain)	*¼ cup (50 mL)	1 cup (250 mL)	8 to 10 min.	2 to 3 min.

* Use a 4 cup (1 L) measuring cup or bowl to prevent boiling over.

Tip

Double the proportions, use container twice the size and increase time to make 2 servings. Refrigerate extra serving and to reheat, microwave at High for 30 to 40 seconds, adding water if necessary for desired consistency.

Variations

1. 2 tbsp. (25 mL) chopped diced fruits, or wheat germ may be added before cooking.

2. Add ¼ tsp. (1 mL) cinnamon.

Quick Microwave
Breakfast Choices

1. Section one-half grapefruit and place in custard cup; top with 1 tsp. (5 mL) brown sugar, honey, maple syrup or marmalade. Microwave at High until hot, about 30 to 45 seconds.

2. Combine ½ cup (125 mL) dried prunes, pears, apricots, peaches or apples with 1 tbsp. (15 mL) water; cover and microwave at High for 1 minute.

3. Top a slice of whole wheat toast with a thin slice of ham and a slice of part-skim mozzarella cheese. Place on paper towel and microwave at High for 20 to 30 seconds or until cheese melts.

4. Spread light cream cheese on whole wheat toast; sprinkle with cinnamon or top with Apple Butter (page 81) or Jane's Apricot Conserve (page 80). Place on paper towel and microwave at High for 10 to 15 seconds or until warm.

5. Make an indentation in the middle of a slice of whole wheat toast. Place on serving plate. Drop a raw egg into the indentation. Pierce the yolk with toothpick or tines of fork. Sprinkle grated part-skim mozzarella cheese on top. Microwave at Medium-High (70%) for 45 to 60 seconds (don't cook it completely). Let stand for 1 to 2 minutes.

Snacks and Totables: grazing goodness

Herbed Focaccia

A popular Italian flat bread, ours is a cinch to make using frozen bread dough. This recipe makes enough to satisfy any team.

¼ cup	finely chopped onion	50 mL
5 tbsp.	finely grated Parmesan cheese, divided	65 mL
1 tsp.	dried rosemary	5 mL
1 lb	whole wheat or white frozen bread dough, thawed	450 g
1 tbsp.	olive oil, divided	15 mL
2 tbsp.	chopped fresh basil OR 2 tsp. (10 mL) dried	25 mL

Makes 8 to 10 servings

1 Serving:
Protein 5 grams
Fat 3 grams
Carbohydrate 28 grams
Calories 159

Method

1. Mix onion, ¼ cup (50 mL) of the cheese and rosemary together.
2. Spread out on work surface. Place dough on top of it; roll dough in onion mixture and push ingredients into dough with hands until incorporated.
3. Put 1 tsp. (5 mL) of the oil in a bowl; add the dough, turning over once or twice to coat with oil; cover with plastic wrap.
4. Turn oven to 200°F (100°C), leave on for 2 minutes and turn off.
5. Place bowl of dough in warm oven and let rise until doubled, about 1½ hours.
6. Roll or pat dough to fit a 15 x 10 inch (40 x 25 cm) non-stick baking sheet.
7. Place dough on it and make several indentations in dough with fingertips to make surface irregular.
8. Brush with remaining oil, sprinkle with basil and remaining cheese.
9. Press the basil into dough.
10. Bake in 400°F (200°C) oven for 15 to 25 minutes or until crisp and browned.
11. Remove from pan; cool slightly and cut into large slices or squares.
12. Serve warm or cool. Focaccia can be frozen for up to 3 months.

Variation

Makes 8 to 10 servings

Tomato Topped Focaccia: After baking focaccia, top with sliced tomatoes, sprinkle with fresh basil, freshly ground pepper and dot with ¼ cup (50 mL) crumbled goat cheese (chèvre). Return to oven until cheese is warm, about 5 minutes.

Bruschetta

½ cup	finely diced tomato	125 mL
1 tbsp.	olive oil	15 mL
1 tsp.	chopped fresh basil leaves OR ¼ tsp. (1 mL) dried	5 mL
1	clove garlic, minced	1
½	green onion, minced	½
1	piece (6 inch/15 cm) French stick (baguette)	1
1 tsp.	grated Parmesan cheese	5 mL

Broiled in minutes, this pizza-like bread makes a splendid appetizer or accompaniment.

Method

1. In a small bowl, mix tomato, oil, basil, garlic and onion together, crushing slightly with a fork.
2. Slice the bread in half lengthwise.
3. Broil or toast cut surface on grill until golden brown, about 1 to 3 minutes.
4. Spoon tomato mixture over toasted bread; press down slightly with a spoon.
5. Sprinkle cheese on top and return to broiler or grill just to warm slightly.
6. To serve, cut each piece in half or quarters.

Makes 2 to 4 servings

1 Serving:
Protein 1 gram
Fat 4 grams
Carbohydrate 6 grams
Calories 64

▦   ▦   ▦   ▦   ▦   ▦   ▦

Intimate Dinner For Two

Bruschetta

Warm Szechuan Chicken Salad (page 124)

Grapefruit Alaska (page 225)

White Bean Hummus

Kidney beans were never more glorious than in this Middle Eastern dip! Serve with Herbed Focaccia (page 86), pita crackers or a variety of raw vegetables for a snack that does a great disappearing act at a gathering of team-mates.

Makes about 2 cups.

1 Serving 2 tbsp/25 mL:
Protein 2 grams
Fat 4 grams
Carbohydrate 5 grams
Calories 64

2	cloves garlic	2
1	19 oz (540 mL) can white kidney beans, drained and rinsed	1
½ cup	tahini	125 mL
2 tbsp.	olive oil	25 mL
¼ cup	lemon juice	50 mL
1 tbsp.	freshly chopped parsley	15 mL
¼ tsp.	salt	1 mL
½ tsp.	ground cumin	2 mL

Method

1. Mince garlic in processor. Add remaining ingredients. Blend until grainy purée forms, scraping down sides of bowl.
2. Transfer to bowl, cover and refrigerate. Can be stored in fridge for up to 3 days.

Variations

Red Pepper Hummus: Add ⅔ cup chopped, drained, roasted red peppers from the jar, and omit the cumin.

Lemony Chickpea Hummus: Substitute 1 can (19 oz/540 mL) chickpeas for the kidney beans, and use the juice of 2 lemons.

Mexican Black Bean Hummus: Substitute 1 can (19 oz/540 mL) black beans for kidney beans and ¼ cup (50 mL) lime juice for the lemon juice. Add ¼ cup (50 mL) freshly chopped coriander and ¾ tsp (4 mL) cayenne.

Tortilla Chips: Stack 3 flour tortillas one on top of the other; cut into six or eight wedges. Repeat with three more tortillas. Spread in a single layer on a baking sheet. Bake in 375°F (190°C) oven for 5 to 8 minutes or until crisp and golden brown. Store in airtight container for up to 1 month.

The longest human-powered sports event is the bicycle race, the Tour de France, which lasts 23 days. In 1926 this was over 3,659 miles, lasting a record 29 days.

Antojitas

¼ cup	light cream cheese	50 mL
½ cup	part-skim mozzarella cheese, grated	125 mL
1 tbsp.	finely diced sweet red pepper or pimento	15 mL
2 tsp.	finely diced pickled jalapeno peppers	10 mL
2 tsp.	finely diced green onion	10 mL
4	7 inch (17 cm) flour tortillas Santa Fe Salsa (page 213)	4

Creamy and spicy, these Mexican tortilla rolls excite the palate. Hot or cold, they are excellent in bite-sized pieces as an hors d'oeuvre or left whole as a totable sandwich for lunch.

Method

1. In a small bowl, stir cream cheese until creamy.
2. Blend in mozzarella cheese, red pepper, jalapeno peppers and green onion.
3. Spread 2 tbsp. (25 mL) of mixture on each tortilla.
4. Roll up jelly-roll style.
5. Wrap and chill for at least 2 hours or up to 3 days.
6. At serving time, if serving as an hors d'oeuvre, cut into 1 inch (2.5 cm) slices.
7. **Bake** in 425°F (220°C) oven for 5 minutes. OR **microwave** at Medium (50%) for 30 to 60 seconds or until hot.
8. Serve with Santa Fe Salsa.

Variation

Add coriander (cilantro) to the cheese mixture. Before serving, alternate slices of avocado and mango on top of the roll for color and flavor. Serve with black beans.

Makes 4 lunch servings or 24 appetizers

1 Appetizer Piece:
Protein 2 grams
Fat 1 gram
Carbohydrate 6 grams
Calories 41

Herbed Pita Crackers

2 tbsp.	olive oil	25 mL
½ tsp.	minced garlic	2 mL
½ tsp.	dried oregano	2 mL
½ tsp.	dried basil	2 mL
2	6 inch (16 cm) whole wheat pitas	2

Great for munching, these low fat crisps are addictive.

Method

1. Combine oil, garlic, oregano and basil.
2. Cut each pita into 8 wedges; separate each wedge into two triangles.
3. Lightly brush the oil mixture on the inside surface.
4. Place brushed side up on ungreased baking sheet.
5. Bake at 350°F (180°C) for 12 to 15 minutes or until crisp and toasted.
6. Serve warm or store in airtight container.

Makes 32 crackers

1 Cracker:
Fat 1 gram
Carbohydrate 2 grams
Calories 17

Creamy Horseradish Topping

Good as a topping for baked potatoes or a dip for crunchy vegetables. For extra zest, add to your roast beef sandwich.

Makes 1/2 cup (125 mL)

1 Tablespoon:
Protein 2 grams
Carbohydrate 0.5 grams
Calories 10

½ cup	2% cottage cheese	125 mL
1 tbsp.	2% milk	15 mL
1 tbsp.	chopped fresh chives	15 mL
1 to 2 tsp.	prepared horseradish	5 to 10 mL
1 tsp.	lemon juice	5 mL

Method
1. In a blender or food processor, combine cottage cheese, milk, chives, horseradish and lemon juice.
2. Process until smooth.
3. Chill until serving time.

Herbed Chèvre

Chèvre is an unripened soft, creamy goat cheese with lower butterfat than many other cheeses. This is a smooth tangy mixture to spread over warm bread as a snack or a "starter."

Makes 1 cup (250 mL)

1 Tablespoon:
Protein 2 grams
Fat 1 gram
Carbohydrate 1 gram
Calories 21

½ cup	creamy goat cheese, at room temperature (about 4 oz/125 g)	125 mL
½ cup	2% cottage cheese	125 mL
1 tbsp.	2% milk	15 mL
1 tbsp.	chopped fresh basil OR 1 tsp. (5 mL) dried	15 mL
1 tsp.	chopped fresh tarragon OR ¼ tsp. (1 mL) dried	5 mL
1	clove garlic, minced	1
1	green onion, chopped	1
¼ tsp.	pepper	1 mL

Method
1. In a blender or food processor, combine goat cheese, cottage cheese, milk, basil, tarragon, garlic, green onion and pepper.
2. Process until smooth.
3. Cover and refrigerate for at least 1 hour or up to 3 days.

Ceviche

8 oz	fresh scallops or red snapper fillets	125 g
¼ cup	orange juice	50 mL
¼ cup	lime juice	50 mL
1 tbsp.	olive oil	15 mL
1	medium tomato, peeled, seeded and diced	1
¼ cup	chopped red onion	50 mL
1 tbsp.	chopped fresh coriander (cilantro) or parsley	15 mL
2 tsp.	chopped pickled jalapeno peppers	10 mL
1	small clove garlic, minced	1
	lettuce leaves	
	lime wedges, coriander (cilantro) or fresh parsley sprigs for garnish	

An appetizer fragrant with citrus and fresh coriander that is low in fat. Set these ingredients to marinate before an afternoon of tennis, and enjoy later.

Method

1. If scallops are large, slice horizontally or cut snapper into ½ inch (1 cm) pieces.
2. In a bowl, mix orange juice, lime juice and oil for marinade.
3. In a shallow glass dish, combine fish, tomato, onion, coriander, peppers and garlic.
4. Pour marinade over fish mixture, stir well and be sure fish is covered with marinade.
5. Cover and refrigerate for at least 2 hours or up to 24 hours.
6. Serve on lettuce leaves garnished with lime wedges and coriander or parsley sprigs.

Makes 4 appetizer servings

1 Appetizer Serving:
Protein 8 grams
Fat 4 grams
Carbohydrate 5 grams
Calories 88

Tip
You can substitute 2 tbsp. (25 mL) chopped canned green chilies and a few drops hot pepper sauce for 2 tsp. (10 mL) chopped pickled jalapeno peppers.

Today's game of tennis has evolved from an 11th century form of French Royal hand-ball called "le jeu de paume." The scoring system may date from the Medieval use of 60 as a base number (we use 100). The term "love" for zero came either from the French, l'oeuf (egg, implying zero), or from the English usage of love as equating nothing ("not for love or money").

Tri-Color Egg Salad

The bright colors of the radishes and green onions add eye-appeal to this crunchy, flavorful favorite.

2	hard-cooked eggs, peeled and chopped	2
¾ cup	2% cottage cheese	175 mL
½ cup	finely chopped radishes	125 mL
1 tbsp.	light mayonnaise	15 mL
1	green onion, chopped	1
2 tsp.	fresh dill OR ½ tsp. (2 mL) dried	10 mL
⅛ tsp.	garlic powder	0.5 mL
⅛ tsp.	salt	0.5 mL
	freshly ground pepper	

Makes 2 servings

1 Serving:
Protein 17 grams
Fat 10 grams
Carbohydrate 4 grams
Calories 174

Method
1. In a small bowl, combine chopped eggs, cottage cheese, radishes, mayonnaise, green onion, dill, garlic powder, salt and pepper to taste.
2. Mix well.
3. Serve immediately or cover and refrigerate for up to 2 days.

Variation
Substitute 1-6 oz (170 g) cake soft drained tofu for the egg. Replace dill and garlic powder with ½ tsp (2 mL) curry powder and ⅛ tsp (0.5 mL) cumin. Serve with whole grain bread.

Tuna Almond Salad

A tasty mixture of fish and grains that can be eaten as a salad or packed into tortillas or pita pockets for a cycling picnic en route.

1	6 oz (170 g) can water-packed tuna, drained and flaked	1
⅔ cup	cooked rice or small pasta shells	150 mL
⅔ cup	2% plain yogurt	150 mL
½ cup	diced sweet red or green pepper	150 mL
¼ cup	toasted slivered almonds or pine nuts	50 mL
¼ cup	diced celery	50 mL
1 tsp.	lemon juice	5 mL
1 tsp.	dried tarragon	5 mL
1	clove garlic, minced	1
	freshly ground pepper	
	lettuce leaves (optional)	

Makes 4 servings

1 Serving:
Protein 19 grams
Fat 5 grams
Carbohydrate 13 grams
Calories 173

Method
1. In a small bowl, combine tuna, rice, yogurt, peppers, almonds, celery, lemon juice, tarragon and garlic; mix well.
2. Season to taste with pepper.
3. Serve on lettuce leaves if using.

Pizza Crisps

1	6 inch (16 cm) whole wheat pita	1
¼ cup	shredded partly skimmed mozzarella cheese	50 mL
⅛ tsp.	dried basil	0.5 mL
⅛ tsp.	dried oregano	0.5 mL
1	green onion, finely diced	1
2	tomato slices	2
	freshly ground pepper	

This fast lunch can be made almost as quickly as lacing up a pair of high tops. It's a pizza that is low in fat yet provides excellent nutrition.

Method
1. Cut around edge of pita to separate into 2 rounds.
2. Place on baking sheet; broil cut side up for 2 to 3 minutes or until lightly golden.
3. In a bowl, combine mozzarella cheese, basil, oregano and onion.
4. Spread cheese over pita halves.
5. Top with tomato slices; sprinkle with pepper to taste.
6. Bake in 400°F (200°C) oven for 5 to 8 minutes or until heated through.

Makes 1 serving

1 Serving:
Protein 12 grams
Fat 1 gram
Carbohydrate 34 grams
Calories 193

Other Quick Toppings
Lightly sautéed vegetables, bottled toppings like roasted red peppers, capers, olives, sundried tomatoes, canned artichokes, chickpeas, anchovies

Running was a part of early Egyptian rituals around 3700 B.C.

Pita Encores

When you're faced with a refrigerator full of lots of little "bits," this sandwich is a refreshing lunch that never hints of "leftovers."

2	5 to 7 inch (12 to 17 cm) whole wheat pitas	2
1 cup	shredded Iceberg lettuce	250 mL
1 cup	grated carrot or zucchini	250 mL
½ cup	diced tomato	125 mL
½ cup	julienned cooked chicken, turkey, ham, cheese or sliced hard cooked egg	125 mL
1	green onion, thinly sliced	1
1 tbsp.	toasted unsalted sunflower seeds (optional)	15 mL
⅓ cup	Herbed Yogurt Dressing (page 112) freshly ground pepper	75 mL

Makes 2 servings

1 Serving:
Protein 22 grams
Fat 12 grams
Carbohydrate 44 grams
Calories 372

Method

1. Warm pitas if desired by wrapping in foil and placing in 200°F (95°C) **oven** for 5 minutes. OR wrap in paper towels and **microwave** at High for 30 seconds.
2. In a medium bowl, combine lettuce, carrot, tomato, chicken, green onion, seeds, if using, and dressing; toss to coat well.
3. Add pepper to taste.
4. Cut pita in half crosswise; gently open each pocket and spoon filling into halves.

To Poach Boneless, Skinless Chicken Breasts: In a shallow microwaveable casserole or plate, place 8 oz. (250 g) boneless, skinless chicken breasts or turkey fillets. Add 1 tbsp. (15 mL) water; cover and microwave at High for 3 to 4 minutes or until no longer pink inside. Let stand for 5 minutes. Cool; cover and chill, or wrap in foil and freeze.

Muffuletta

2	large whole wheat rolls	2
1	tomato, seeded and finely chopped	1
½ cup	canned artichoke hearts, drained and chopped	125 mL
¼ cup	finely diced sweet green pepper	50 mL
2 tbsp.	chopped green onion	25 mL
1 tbsp.	chopped capers	15 mL
¼ tsp.	pepper	1 mL
⅛ tsp.	salt	0.5 mL
⅛ tsp.	dried oregano (optional)	0.5 mL
⅛ tsp.	dried basil (optional)	0.5 mL
¼ cup	grated Parmesan cheese	50 mL
1 tsp.	olive oil	5 mL
1	part–skim mozzarella cheese slice, halved	1

We've adapted this sophisticated New Orleans-style sandwich in order to reduce the fat yet retain all the sunny goodness in its taste.

Method

1. Cut tops off rolls. Scoop out crumbs leaving a ½ inch (1 cm) shell.
2. In a small bowl break bread crumbs into smaller pieces; add tomatoes, artichokes, peppers, onion, capers, pepper, salt, oregano, basil and Parmesan cheese.
3. Brush inside of rolls with olive oil.
4. Place a slice of mozzarella cheese in bottom half of each roll.
5. Spoon vegetable mixture on top of cheese; replace top.
6. Wrap and chill for up to 4 hours.
7. Cut crosswise to serve.

Makes 2 servings

1 Serving:
Protein 15 grams
Fat 10 grams
Carbohydrate 47 grams
Calories 338

Patsy's Celery Root Remoulade

Our friend Patsy Jamieson likes to serve this flavorful fall vegetable as a salad on a bed of lettuce topped with minced parsley. It is equally good teamed up with lean turkey for a lunchtime sandwich.

Makes 2 cups (500 mL)

1 Cup:
Protein 3 grams
Fat 2.5 grams
Carbohydrate 11 grams
Calories 79

2 tbsp.	2% plain yogurt	25 mL
1 to 2 tbsp.	Dijon mustard	15 mL to 25 mL
1 tbsp.	light mayonnaise	15 mL
1 tsp.	2% milk	5 mL
⅛ tsp.	salt	0.5 mL
	freshly ground pepper	
2 cups	peeled and grated celery root	500 mL
	minced fresh parsley (optional)	

Method

1. In a small bowl, combine yogurt, mustard, mayonnaise, milk, salt and pepper to taste; mix well.
2. Stir in celery root.
3. Sprinkle parsley, if using, over top.

Celeriac (celery root or knob celery) resembles the homely turnip. It is not the root of the celery plant familiar to all crudite fans, but does impart a strong celery flavor.

Pasta with Ceci (page 104)
Carrot Soup (page 110)

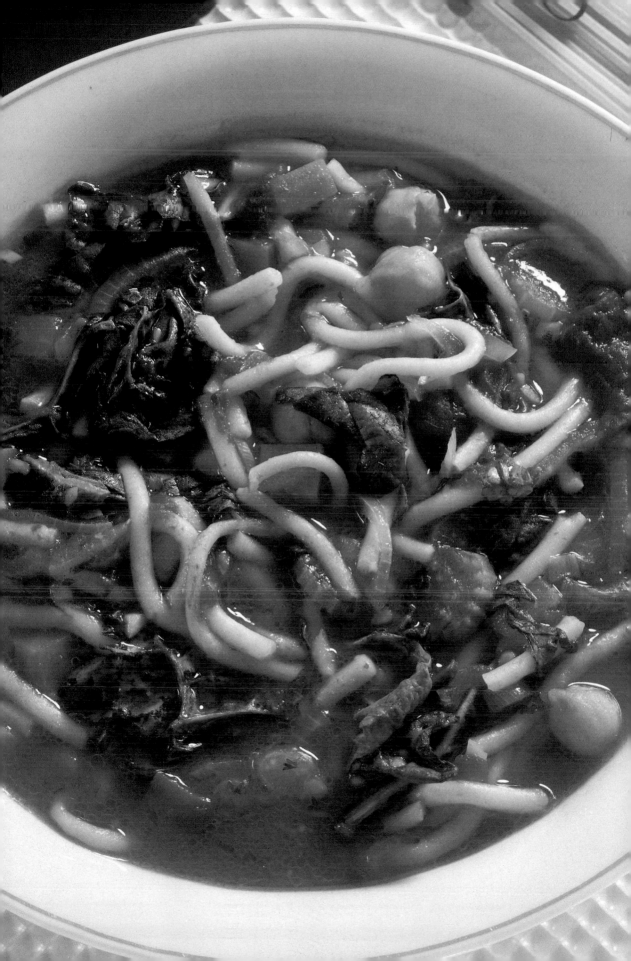

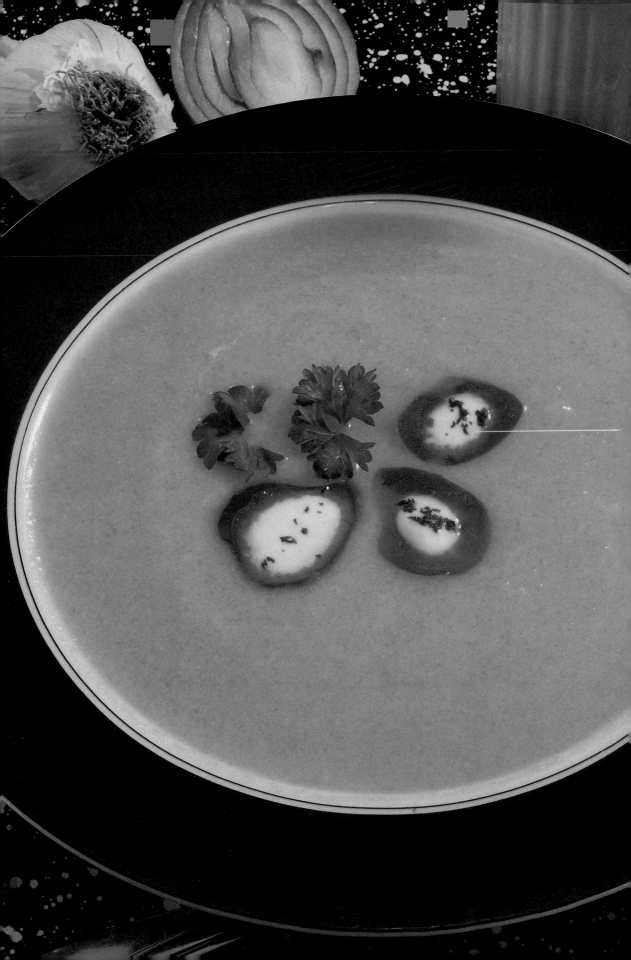

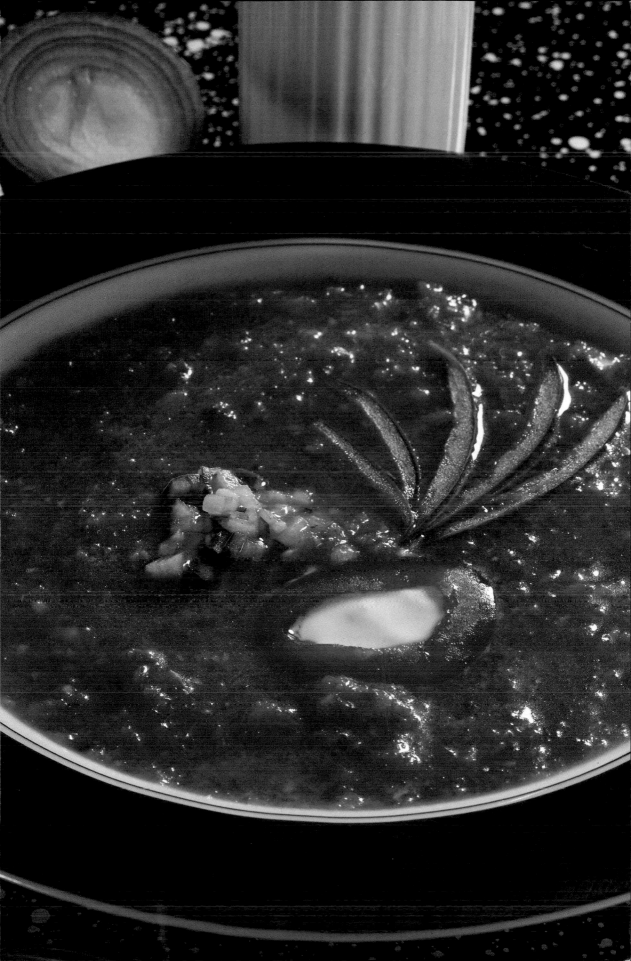

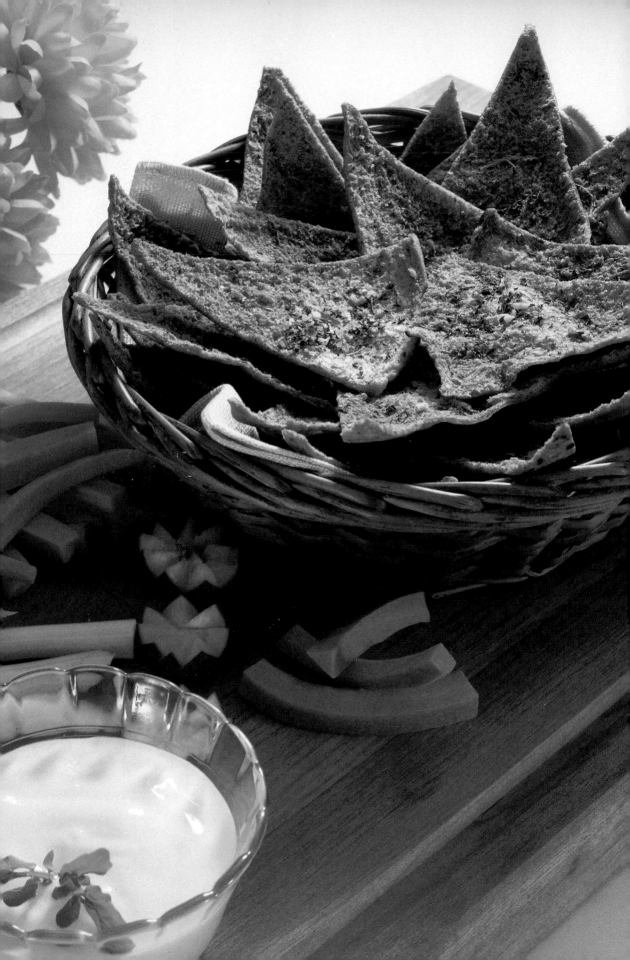

Salmon Pâté

1	7.75 oz (220 g) can salmon, drained	1
¼ cup	light cream cheese, softened	50 mL
¼ tsp.	horseradish	1 mL
	capers (optional)	

Method
1. In a small bowl, flake salmon and mash bones with fork.
2. Blend cream cheese and horseradish into salmon.

Variations
Mackerel: Substitute 1 can (6 ½ oz/184 g) mackerel packed in tomato sauce for salmon. Do not drain mackerel and omit horseradish.

Sardine: Substitute 2 cans (100 g) sardines packed in water, drained, for salmon. Omit horseradish. Add 1 tbsp. (15 mL) Dijon mustard and 1 tbsp. (15 mL) chopped capers.

Packed Lunch Tips
▦ Save time and make lots of sandwiches at one time and then freeze sandwiches.
▦ When preparing sandwiches before freezing, spread bread right to crusts with butter or light cream cheese.
▦ Firm cheese slices such as part-skim mozzarella and cold cooked roast beef, pork, ham or chicken can be successfully frozen.
▦ The salmon, mackerel and sardine fillings can also be successfully frozen.
▦ Avoid freezing hard-cooked egg or mayonnaise fillings.
▦ Pack lettuce, sprouts, tomatoes and cucumbers separately – add to sandwiches at serving time.

This spread freezes well for sandwiches on the go, or is elegant enough to serve to friends as an hors d'oeuvre with crackers. Canned salmon is an excellent source of calcium and omega-3-fatty acids.

Makes enough filling for 5 sandwiches

1 Sandwich Filling:
Protein 10 grams
Fat 7 grams
Calories 103

Gazpacho (page 99)
Herbed Pita Crackers (page 89)

Chili Munch

After a tough game of squash or racquetball, this mixture is addictive as the perfect partner to a celebratory beer. Enjoy as a snack any time.

2	egg whites	2
1 tbsp.	chili powder	15 mL
½ tsp.	ground cumin	2 mL
½ tsp.	garlic powder	2 mL
1 cup	toasted oat cereal (e.g., Cheerios®)	250 mL
1 cup	corn bran cereal	250 mL
1 cup	whole wheat cereal squares (e.g., Shreddies®)	250 mL
1 cup	pumpkin (pepita) seeds	250 mL
1 cup	unblanched almonds	250 mL
⅔ cup	raisins	150 mL

Makes about 5 cups (1.25 L)

1 Cup:
Protein 17 grams
Fat 29 grams
Carbohydrate 47 grams
Calories 517

Method

1. In a large bowl, beat egg white until foamy and soft peaks form.
2. Fold chili powder, cumin and garlic powder into egg whites.
3. Add cereals, pumpkin seeds and almonds; stir to coat well.
4. Spread on non-stick baking sheet. Bake in 300°F (150°C) oven for 10 to 12 minutes or until crisp and lightly browned, stirring every 5 minutes.
5. Add raisins and cool.
6. Store in airtight containers or plastic bags.

Indian Variation
Substitute curry powder for chili powder and ⅛ tsp. (0.5 mL) cayenne powder for cumin in recipe and substitute unsweetened coarsely flaked coconut for raisins.

Sweet Tooth Variation
Omit chili, cumin and garlic powder. Use 2 tbsp. (25 mL) brown sugar, 1 tsp. (5 mL) cinnamon, 1 tsp. (5 mL) nutmeg. Substitute sliced dried apples for raisins.

Super Fit Soups

Gazpacho

2	large tomatoes, peeled and coarsely chopped	2
½ cup	peeled and sliced English cucumber	125 mL
¼ cup	sliced onion	50 mL
¼ cup	coarsely chopped green pepper	50 mL
1	small clove garlic, minced	1
¼ cup	water	50 mL
2 tbsp.	red wine vinegar	25 mL
1 tbsp.	olive oil	15 mL
¼ tsp.	salt	1 mL
¼ tsp.	paprika	1 mL
	freshly ground pepper	
	2% plain yogurt, finely diced cucumber, green pepper and/or onion for garnishes	

A chunky, fresh vegetable soup laced with the flavors of onion and garlic for a cool, refreshing lunch. Packed with vitamin C, this soup can help rehydrate tired cyclists on an all-day outing.

Method

1. In a large bowl, combine tomatoes, cucumber, onion, green pepper, garlic, water, vinegar, oil, salt, paprika and pepper to taste.
2. Stir to mix well; pour into blender or food processor. Turn motor on and off (pushing vegetables down sides as needed) just until vegetables are coarsely chopped but not puréed.
3. Pour into a bowl or jar; cover and refrigerate for ½ hour or overnight.
4. To serve, top with dollop of yogurt and sprinkle diced cucumber, green pepper and/or onion.

Makes 2 servings

1 Serving:
Protein 2 grams
Fat 7 grams
Carbohydrate 14 grams
Calories 127

Fresh Tomato Basil Soup

The vigorous flavors of this summer herb and vegetable soup complement any sport.

1	small leek, white part only	1
1 tsp.	vegetable oil	10 mL
1	clove garlic, minced	1
1	28 oz (796 mL) can tomatoes OR 3 cups (750 mL) fresh, peeled and diced	1
1 tbsp.	chopped fresh basil OR 1 tsp (5 mL) dried	15 mL
1 tsp.	chicken stock granules freshly ground pepper 2% plain yogurt for garnish fresh basil leaves for garnish	5 mL

Makes 2 to 3 servings

1 Serving:
Protein 2.5 grams
Fat 3 grams
Carbohydrate 13 grams
Calories 89

Method

1. Cut leek in half lengthwise and wash well to remove grit; slice.
2. In a large non-stick saucepan, heat oil over medium heat. Add leek and garlic; sauté for 4 to 5 minutes or until vegetables are tender.
3. Add tomatoes, basil, chicken stock granules and pepper to taste; cover and bring to boil.
4. Reduce heat and simmer for 10 to 15 minutes.
5. Remove from heat. Purée in blender or food processor and return to saucepan. Heat until hot.
6. Garnish each bowl with swirl of yogurt and fresh basil.

Cocooning Menu

Fresh Tomato Basil Soup

Comfort Supper (page 136)

Technicolor Coleslaw (page 129)

Fruit Crisp (page 236)

Cucumber Frappé

½	English cucumber OR 1 field cucumber	½	
2 cups	2% plain yogurt	500 mL	
1	clove garlic, minced	1	
1 tbsp.	chicken stock granules	15 mL	
1 tsp.	minced fresh dill OR ¼ tsp. (1 mL) dried dillweed		
¼ tsp.	ground white pepper fresh dill sprigs for garnish	1 mL	

Tart and refreshing, this no-cook soup goes anywhere in a thermos and is simple to make at the touch of a button.

Method

1. Peel about one half of the cucumber leaving some skin on; cut into 1 inch (2.5 cm) pieces.
2. In a blender or food processor, combine cucumber, yogurt, garlic, chicken stock granules, minced dill and pepper; process until completely puréed.
3. Chill for ½ hour or overnight.
4. Garnish each portion with dill sprigs.

Makes 4 servings

1 Serving:
Protein 7 grams
Fat 2 grams
Carbohydrate 10 grams
Calories 86

▓   ▓   ▓   ▓   ▓   ▓   ▓

Entertaining Menu

Cucumber Frappé

Lamb Tandoori (page 187)

Apple Chutney (page 216)

Basmati Rice

Braised Carrots and Parsnips (page 153)

Raspberry Yogurt Mousse (page 229)

Mushroom Barley Soup

Great tasting, this rich brown soup is hearty with mushrooms and barley and fragrant with fresh dill. Perfect for warming up after a morning on the ski trails.

4 cups	beef stock	1 L
¼ cup	uncooked barley	50 mL
1 tbsp.	vegetable oil	15 mL
½ cup	chopped onion	125 mL
⅓ cup	chopped celery	75 mL
2	cloves garlic, minced	2
4 cups	sliced fresh mushrooms (about 1 lb/500 g)	1 L
2 tbsp.	dry vermouth or sherry	25 mL
2 tbsp.	fresh dill	25 mL
⅛ tsp.	salt	0.5 mL
	freshly ground pepper	

Makes 4 to 5 servings

1 Serving:
Protein 4 grams
Fat 3 grams
Carbohydrate 14 grams
Calories 99

Method

1. In a large saucepan, bring stock to boil; stir in barley, reduce heat and simmer for 45 to 60 minutes or until barley is tender.
2. In non-stick skillet, heat oil over medium heat. Add onion, celery and garlic; sauté for 2 to 3 minutes or until softened.
3. Add mushrooms and vermouth; stir and cook for 2 to 3 minutes or until mushrooms are tender.
4. Add to barley mixture; heat through.
5. Stir in dill; season with salt and pepper.
6. As soup stands barley absorbs liquid; add water or stock to adjust to desired consistency.

Portuguese Kale and Potato Soup

2 tsp.	olive oil	10 mL
1	clove garlic, minced	1
1	small onion, chopped	1
1	parsnip, chopped	1
1	large baking potato, peeled and chopped	1
2 cups	chicken stock or vegetable stock	500 mL
8 oz	low-fat kielbasa sausage, chopped	250 g
½ tsp.	pepper	2 mL
4 cups	kale, stems discarded, well rinsed and shredded	1 L

Whether it's winter outside, or you just want the warm comfort of a hearty soup within you, this combination of dark greens, low-fat protein and lip-smacking flavor is unbeatable.

Method

1. Heat the oil in a medium saucepan over medium-low heat. Add garlic, onion and parsnip, stirring until softened, about 5 minutes.
2. Add the baking potato, chicken stock and 2 cups water. Bring to a boil, and simmer, covered, 10 to 15 minutes, or until the potato is tender.
3. Add the sausage, kale and pepper. Simmer for 10 minutes or until kale is bright green and tender.

Makes about 6 cups, 4 to 6 servings

1 Serving:
Protein 9 grams
Fat 7 grams
Carbohydrate 25 grams
Calories 199

Pasta with Ceci

This hearty, satisfying Italian soup combines all four food groups for a perfectly balanced meal. Easily transported in a thermos, it can be a quick nutritious lunch after a midday workout.

1 tbsp.	olive oil	15 mL
½ cup	chopped onion	125 mL
½ cup	chopped celery	125 mL
2	cloves garlic, minced	2
1 cup	finely diced carrots	250 mL
1	28 oz (796 mL) can tomatoes	1
4 cups	water	1 L
1 tsp.	dried oregano	5 mL
½ tsp.	dried thyme	2 mL
¼ tsp.	freshly ground pepper	1 mL
¼ tsp.	salt	1 mL
4 oz	uncooked, broken spaghetti	125 g
1	19 oz (540 mL) can chickpeas, undrained	1
5 cups	washed spinach or Swiss chard	1.25 L
¼ cup	grated Parmesan cheese	50 mL

Method

1. In a large non-stick saucepan, heat oil over medium heat. Add onion, celery and garlic; sauté for 2 to 3 minutes or until onion has softened.
2. Add carrots, tomatoes, water, oregano, thyme, pepper and salt. Cover and bring to boil.
3. Reduce heat and simmer for 30 to 40 minutes or until carrot is almost cooked.
4. Return to boil, add spaghetti and liquid from chickpeas and simmer for 5 to 10 minutes, stirring occasionally or until spaghetti is almost cooked.
5. Remove stems from spinach and tear into large pieces. Stir into soup along with chickpeas. Heat until hot and spinach has wilted.
6. Top each serving with Parmesan cheese.

Makes 4 to 6 servings

1 Serving:
Protein 10 grams
Fat 5 grams
Carbohydrate 36 grams
Calories 229

Swimming was first a survival skill among the ancient Egyptians, Greeks and Romans, not a sport. Japan issued an Imperial decree in the early 1600s, ordering swimming to be part of the educational curriculum, thus initiating swimming meets. Competitive swimming did not reach Europe and Great Britain for another two centuries.

Hot and Sour Soup

4 oz	boneless, skinless chicken breast, or pork tenderloin	125 mL
1 tbsp.	soy sauce	15 mL
3 to 4	dried Chinese mushrooms (about ½ oz/14 g)	3 to 4
3 cups	chicken stock	750 mL
¼ cup	fresh, sliced mushrooms, such as oyster	125 mL
2 tbsp.	rice or white wine vinegar	25 mL
½ to 1 tsp.	white pepper	2 to 5 mL
1 tbsp.	cornstarch	15 mL
4 oz	diced tofu (about ½ cup/125 mL)	125 g
1 tsp.	sesame oil	5 mL
1	egg white	1
	chopped green onion for garnish	

The title says it all! Broth as spicy as your palate can stand plus high protein tofu for a soup to sustain your sports.

Method

1. Slice chicken in very thin strips; combine with soy sauce and refrigerate for 30 minutes.
2. Soak dried mushrooms in warm water for 30 minutes; drain.
3. Cut off and discard any tough stem ends, cut in half and thinly slice.
4. In a large saucepan, bring chicken stock to boil. Add chicken, Chinese mushrooms, fresh mushrooms, vinegar and pepper to taste; simmer covered for 10 minutes.
5. Mix cornstarch with 2 tbsp. (25 mL) water and stir into soup; bring to boil and cook stirring constantly for 2 to 3 minutes.
6. Add tofu and sesame oil.
7. Just before serving, beat egg white with 1 tbsp. (15 mL) water; add to hot soup in a thin stream beating constantly.
8. Garnish individual servings with green onion.

Makes 2 to 3 servings

1 Serving:
Protein 13 grams
Fat 4 grams
Carbohydrate 5 grams
Calories 108

Spring Soup

An unusual combination of
spring vegetables blends
together for a smooth fresh
green soup, subtly laced
with tarragon.

3 cups	chicken stock	750 mL
1 cup	fresh or frozen green beans	250 mL
⅓ cup	chopped onion	75 mL
2 tbsp.	long-grain rice	25 mL
1½ cups	shredded lettuce	375 mL
1 cup	frozen green peas	250 mL
½ tsp.	dried tarragon	2 mL
⅛ tsp.	salt	0.5 mL
	freshly ground pepper	
	2% plain yogurt for garnish	

**Makes 3 to 4
servings**

1 Serving:
Protein 3 grams
Carbohydrate 14 grams
Calories 68
Fat trace

Method

1. In a large saucepan, combine chicken stock, beans, onion and rice; bring to boil.
2. Cover and reduce heat to medium and cook for 20 to 25 minutes or until beans and rice are tender.
3. Add lettuce and cook for 5 minutes.
4. Add peas and heat to thaw.
5. Add tarragon and salt.
6. Purée in blender or food processor.
7. Taste and adjust seasoning with pepper.
8. Garnish each bowl with a swirl of yogurt.

Creamy Golden Soup

1	2 lb (500 g) acorn or butternut squash, chopped (about 2½ cups/625 mL)	1
2 cups	chicken stock	500 mL
½ cup	finely chopped onion	125 mL
1	clove garlic, minced	1
½ cup	2% milk	125 mL
1½ tbsp.	frozen orange juice concentrate, thawed	20 mL
½ tsp.	ground ginger	2 mL
⅛ tsp.	pepper	0.5 mL
	2% plain yogurt for garnish	
	minced fresh parsley for garnish	

Velvety on the tongue, this orange-flavored squash soup has just the right touch of ginger.

Method
1. Peel, seed and coarsely chop squash.
2. In a large saucepan, combine squash, chicken stock, onion and garlic; bring to boil.
3. Reduce heat and simmer covered until tender, 25 to 30 minutes.
4. Purée in blender or food processor. Stir in milk, orange juice, ginger and pepper.
5. Return to saucepan and heat until hot.
6. Garnish with a swirl of yogurt and/or minced parsley.

Microwave Method
1. Pierce whole squash several times; microwave at High for 4 to 5 minutes to soften.
2. Cut in half; scoop out the seeds. Peel and coarsely chop.
3. In a 2 qt. (2 L) microwaveable container combine squash, chicken stock, onion and garlic; cover and microwave at High for 8 minutes.
4. Stir; microwave covered at High for 8 to 12 minutes or until tender.
5. Purée in blender or food processor. Stir in milk, orange juice, ginger and pepper.
6. Return to container and microwave at High until hot.

Makes 4 to 6 servings

1 Serving:
Protein 2 grams
Fat 0.5 gram
Carbohydrate 12 grams
Calories 60

Mid-Eastern Lentil Soup

Fragrant with a nice balance of cumin and coriander, this soup is hearty enough for a main dish. The red lentils cook as quickly as rice and are important to every athlete as an excellent source of protein and complex carbohydrates.

Makes 2 to 3 servings

1 Serving:
Protein 6 grams
Fat 4 grams
Carbohydrate 25 grams
Calories 160

1 tbsp.	olive oil	15 mL
½ cup	chopped onion	125 mL
½ cup	chopped celery	125 mL
1	clove garlic, minced	1
½ cup	red lentils	125 mL
2 cups	chicken stock	500 mL
½ cup	grated carrot	125 mL
½ cup	chopped apple	125 mL
¾ tsp.	ground cumin	4 mL
¾ tsp.	ground coriander (cilantro)	4 mL
2 tbsp.	chopped fresh parsley	25 mL
¼ tsp.	salt	1 mL
	whole wheat croutons for garnish	

Method

1. In a medium non-stick saucepan, heat oil over medium heat. Add onion, celery and garlic; sauté for 2 to 3 minutes or until softened.
2. Rinse lentils under running water.
3. Add lentils to saucepan along with chicken stock; cover and bring to boil.
4. Reduce heat and simmer for 20 minutes.
5. Add carrot, apple, cumin and coriander; simmer for 10 minutes longer or until lentils are tender.
6. Add parsley. Taste and add salt.
7. Garnish with whole wheat croutons.

Whole Wheat Croutons: Place 2 cups (500 mL) whole wheat bread cubes in a shallow baking dish. **Bake** in 300°F (150°C) oven until crisp and toasted. OR **microwave** at High for 3 to 4 minutes, stirring once, or until crisp.

Seafood and Soba Noodle Soup

2 oz	soba noodles (buckwheat), broken in half	60 g
4 cups	chicken or fish stock	1 L
½ cup	julienned carrot (about ½ a carrot)	125 mL
1 cup	shitake, oyster or enoki mushrooms thinly sliced	250 mL
½ cup	diagonally sliced snow peas	125 mL
4 tsp.	finely minced gingerroot	20 mL
2	cloves garlic, minced	2
1 tbsp.	soy sauce or tamari	15 mL
1 tbsp.	rice wine vinegar	15 mL
4 oz	medium frozen shrimp or scallops, thawed	125 g
	chopped green onion for garnish	

Method

1. In a large pot of boiling water, cook noodles just until tender but firm, about 5 minutes (or according to package directions). Drain.
2. Meanwhile, in a medium saucepan bring stock to boil. Add carrots; cook for 2 to 3 minutes.
3. Add mushrooms, snow peas, ginger, garlic, soy sauce and vinegar; simmer for about 3 minutes or until vegetables are tender-crisp.
4. Add shrimp and cook just until shrimp turns pink, about 3 minutes.
5. Divide noodles into individual bowls and ladle broth mixture over top.
6. Garnish with chopped green onion.

A delicate Oriental flavor makes this elegant soup especially enjoyable alone or when entertaining guests. After a strenuous day on the court, this appealing first course will take the edge off a sharp appetite.

Makes 3 to 4 servings

1 Serving:
Protein 10 grams
Carbohydrate 16 grams
Calories 113
Fat 1 gram

Made from buckwheat flour, Japanese soba noodles contain protein and other nutrients which make this soup extra nourishing. Of all the grains, buckwheat is unique as the premier source of available protein.

Carrot Soup

Hot or cold, this soup is a beta-carotene booster.

1 tbsp.	olive oil	15 mL
1½ cups	chopped carrot	375 mL
¾ cup	chopped celery	175 mL
½ cup	chopped onion	125 mL
2 cups	chicken stock	500 mL
¾ cup	dry white wine	175 mL
1 tbsp.	frozen orange juice concentrate, thawed	15 mL
1 tsp.	curry powder	5 mL
½ tsp.	ground nutmeg	2 mL
1 cup	buttermilk	250 mL
	minced parsley for garnish	

Makes 4 servings

1 Serving:
Protein 3 grams
Fat 3 grams
Carbohydrate 13 grams
Calories 91

Method

1. In a large non-stick saucepan, heat oil over medium heat. Add carrots, celery and onion; sauté for 4 to 5 minutes or until softened.
2. Add chicken stock, wine, orange juice concentrate, curry and nutmeg.
3. Bring to boil; reduce heat and simmer covered for about 40 minutes or until carrot is tender.
4. Remove from heat and purée in a blender or food processor.
5. Return to saucepan and add buttermilk. Heat until hot.
6. Serve hot or chilled.
7. Garnish each serving with minced parsley.

Salads: for a strong start and a record finish

Light Vinaigrette

½ cup	chicken stock	125 mL
3 tbsp.	vegetable oil	50 mL
3 tbsp.	white wine vinegar	50 mL
1 tbsp.	Dijon mustard	15 mL
¼ tsp.	freshly ground pepper	1 mL
⅛ tsp.	salt	0.5 mL

Enjoy this low calorie, low fat version of a basic dressing.

Method
1. In a jar, combine chicken stock, oil, vinegar, mustard, pepper and salt; secure lid and shake to mix well.
2. Store in refrigerator for up to 1 week.

Suggestion
Liven up your salad bowl with a variety of salad greens. Try Bibb lettuce, Lamb's lettuce, radicchio, romaine lettuce, Belgian endive, arugula, watercress and dandelion greens.

Makes about 3/4 cup (175 mL)

1 Tablespoon:
Fat 4 grams
Calories 36

Blue Cheese Dressing

½ cup	2% plain yogurt	125 mL
¼ cup	crumbled blue cheese	50 mL
1 tbsp.	light mayonnaise	15 mL
1	small clove garlic, chopped	1

A lighter version of the classic favorite.

Method
1. In a blender, combine yogurt, cheese, mayonnaise and garlic; blend until smooth.
2. Cover and store in refrigerator for up to 3 days.

Makes 3/4 cup (175 mL)

1 Tablespoon:
Protein 1 gram
Fat 1 gram
Carbohydrate 1 gram
Calories 17

Ranch-Style Buttermilk Dressing

Tastes better (we think) and is lower in both sodium and calories than the commercial preparations.

⅓ cup	buttermilk	75 mL
2 tbsp.	light mayonnaise	25 mL
1 tbsp.	chopped fresh dill OR 1 tsp. (5 mL) dried	15 mL
½ tsp.	Dijon mustard	2 mL
¼ tsp.	salt	1 mL
⅛ tsp.	freshly ground pepper	0.5 mL
½	clove garlic, minced	½

Makes 1/2 cup (125 mL)

2 Tablespoons:
Protein 0.5 gram
Fat 2.0 grams
Carbohydrate 0.5 gram
Calories 22

Method

1. In a bowl or jar, combine buttermilk, mayonnaise, dill, mustard, salt, pepper and garlic; shake or whisk until smooth.
2. Cover and store in refrigerator for up to 4 days.

Herbed Yogurt Dressing

A creamy dressing reduced in fat that is delicious enough for everyday use.

¼ cup	2% plain yogurt	50 mL
2 tbsp.	olive oil	25 mL
1 tbsp.	lemon juice	15 mL
¼ tsp.	dried oregano	2 mL
¼ tsp.	dried basil	2 mL
¼ tsp.	salt	2 mL
⅛ tsp.	garlic powder	1 mL
	freshly ground pepper	

Makes 1/2 cup (125 mL)

1 Tablespoon:
Fat 3 grams
Carbohydrate 0.5 gram
Calories 29

Method

1. In a bowl or jar, combine yogurt, oil, lemon juice, oregano, basil, salt, garlic powder and pepper to taste; secure lid and shake to mix well.
2. Store in refrigerator for up to 3 days.

Herbed Vinegar: In a small stainless steel saucepan, heat 2 cups (500 mL) cider, white wine or white vinegar but do not boil; pour over ½ cup (125 mL) coarsely chopped or torn herbs (e.g., tarragon, dill, basil, oregano) in a bowl or glass jar. Let stand for 1 to 2 weeks. Strain and bottle. Add a fresh sprig of the herb for appearance if desired.

Light Caesar-Style Dressing

⅓ cup	Light Vinaigrette (page 111)	75 mL
¼ cup	grated Parmesan cheese	50 mL
2 tbsp.	2% plain yogurt	25 mL
1 tbsp.	red wine vinegar	15 mL
1 to 2	cloves garlic, minced	1 to 2
¼ to ½ tsp.	Dijon mustard	1 to 2 mL

Method
1. In a jar, combine Light Vinaigrette, cheese, yogurt, vinegar, garlic and mustard; secure lid and shake to mix well.
2. Store in refrigerator for up to 3 days.

Serving Suggestion
Great Caesar for Two: Rub cut garlic clove over salad bowl. Add 4 cups (1 L) bite-sized pieces of romaine lettuce, ¼ cup (50 mL) Light Caesar-Style Dressing and 2 tbsp. (25 mL) Parmesan cheese; toss. Season with lots of freshly ground pepper and top with Whole Wheat Croutons (page 108).

Adapted in response to today's health concerns, this perennial favorite delivers all the taste with much less fat and calories

Makes about 1/2 cup (125 mL)

1 Tablespoon:
Protein 1 gram
Fat 3 grams
Calories 31

Tri-Color Pepper Salad

1½ cups	large chunks mixed sweet yellow, red, green or purple peppers	375 mL
¼ cup	sliced red or Spanish onion	50 mL
1 tbsp.	red wine vinegar	15 mL
1 tbsp.	olive oil	15 mL
½ tsp.	fresh oregano OR ⅛ tsp. (0.5 mL) dried	2 mL
⅛ tsp.	salt	0.5 mL
	freshly ground pepper	

Method
1. In a large bowl, toss peppers, onion, vinegar, oil, oregano, salt and pepper; marinate at room temperature for 30 minutes or refrigerate overnight.

Lively to the eye and the palate, this salad is a great accompaniment to barbecued burgers. Peppers are an excellent source of vitamin C and beta-carotene.

Makes 2 servings

1 Serving:
Fat 7 grams
Carbohydrate 3 Grams
Calories 75

The longest annual walking event is the Paris-Colmar event, which is 322 miles.

Soba Noodle Salad

Crisp, colorful vegetables
mixed with a delicate
Oriental dressing for a truly
sensational salad.

2 tbsp.	soy sauce	25 mL
1 tbsp.	rice vinegar	15 mL
1 tbsp.	olive oil	15 mL
1 tsp.	minced fresh gingerroot	5 mL
1	small clove garlic, minced	1
4 oz	soba noodles (buckwheat)	125 g
1 cup	snow peas	250 mL
½ cup	julienned sweet red pepper	125 mL
½ cup	thinly sliced celery	125 mL
½ cup	thinly sliced Chinese cabbage (Nappa)	125 mL
¼ cup	thinly sliced canned water chestnuts	50 mL
1	green onion, sliced	1

Method

1. In a small bowl, mix soy sauce, vinegar, oil, ginger and garlic together and set aside.
2. In a large saucepan of boiling water, cook noodles for 3 to 6 minutes or just until tender but still firm.
3. Drain; chill in cold water for up to 1 hour.
4. Cut any large snow peas in half and blanch in boiling water for 1 minute, drain and plunge into cold water.
5. Drain noodles and snow peas; combine with red pepper, celery, cabbage and water chestnuts.
6. Pour soy sauce mixture on top; toss to coat well.
7. Sprinkle green onion on top and serve.

Variation
Drain ¼ lb (125 g) firm tofu and cut into ½ inch cubes. In a medium-sized skillet, heat 1 tbsp. (15 mL) vegetable oil over high heat. Sauté tofu until browned. Serve over noodle salad and garnish with sesame seeds.

Makes 2 servings

1 Serving:
Protein 11 grams
Fat 7 grams
Carbohydrate 58 grams
Calories 339

Niçoise Pasta Salad

1½ cups	rotini pasta (about 4 oz/125 g)	375 mL
1 cup	halved green beans	250 mL
4	black olives, sliced	4
4	green onions, sliced	4
2	hard-cooked eggs, cut in wedges	2
1	medium tomato, cut into eighths	1
1	sweet red or green pepper, thinly sliced	1
2 tbsp.	capers	25 mL
1	6 oz (170 g) can of tuna, packed in water, drained	1
¼ cup	white wine vinegar	50 mL
2 tbsp.	olive oil	25 mL
4 tsp.	Dijon mustard	20 mL
1 to 2	cloves garlic, minced	1 to 2
¼ tsp.	salt	1 mL
	freshly ground pepper	

Method

1. In a large pot of boiling water, cook pasta until tender but firm; drain and cool under running water; drain and transfer to large bowl.
2. Steam beans for 2 to 3 minutes or until tender-crisp; plunge into cold water to cool; drain.
3. Add to pasta, along with olives, onions, eggs, tomato, pepper and capers.
4. Coarsely flake tuna and add to pasta mixture.
5. Mix vinegar, oil, mustard, garlic, salt and pepper.
6. Pour over pasta mixture. Serve immediately or cover and refrigerate for up to 8 hours.

After a day of sun and windsurfing, this is a satisfying dinner on a summer evening. Our salad with its Mediterranean flavors is also a good source of low fat protein and complex carbohydrates.

Makes 3 to 4 servings

1 Serving:
Protein 20 grams
Fat 8 grams
Carbohydrate 19 grams
Calories 228

Watercress and Beets Vinaigrette

This classic, elegant salad is a truly winning first course. One cup (250 mL) drained, canned beets can be substituted for fresh cooked beets.

Makes 2 to 3 servings

1 Serving:
Protein 6 grams
Fat 8 grams
Carbohydrate 13 grams
Calories 148

2	medium beets	2
¼ cup	water	50 mL
⅓ cup	Light Vinaigrette (page 111)	75 mL
2 heads	Belgian endive, separated into leaves	2 heads
2 cups	watercress leaves, coarse stems removed	500 mL
1	hard-cooked egg, diced for garnish	1

Microwave Method

1. In a 4 cup (1 L) microwaveable casserole, combine beets with water; cover and microwave at High for 8 to 10 minutes or until tender.
2. Drain and let stand until cool enough to handle.
3. Peel and cut into julienne strips.
4. Spoon 2 tbsp. (25 mL) of Light Vinaigrette over beets; set aside.
5. Arrange Belgian endive leaves around the outside of a serving plate.
6. Place watercress in the center of plate; arrange beets on top.
7. Drizzle remaining dressing over endive and watercress.
8. Garnish with diced egg.

Angel Hair Pasta with Lemon and Dill

3 tbsp.	lemon juice	50 mL
2 tbsp.	olive oil	25 mL
1 tsp.	grated lemon rind	5 mL
1 tsp.	Dijon mustard	5 mL
1	clove garlic, minced	1
¼ tsp.	salt	1 mL
	freshly ground pepper	
1 cup	broccoli florets	250 mL
1	broccoli stem	1
1 cup	julienned carrots	250 mL
4 oz	angel hair pasta	125 g
⅓ cup	ricotta cheese	75 mL
1 tbsp.	minced fresh dill	15 mL
	julienned lemon rind for garnish	

The fresh flavor of dill marries happily with this tangy, creamy dressing – tossed quickly with pasta and vegetables. An excellent main dish salad for athletes who are carbohydrate loading for their sport.

Method

1. In a small bowl, mix lemon juice, olive oil, lemon rind, mustard, garlic, salt and pepper; set aside.
2. Cut broccoli florets into narrow thin slices.
3. Peel woody outer layers off broccoli stem; cut into julienne strips.
4. Steam strips of broccoli stem and carrot in vegetable steamer over boiling water for 2 minutes; add broccoli florets and steam for 3 minutes longer or until tender-crisp.
5. Drain and plunge into cold water to cool; drain well.
6. Cook pasta until tender but firm; cool under cold running water; drain well and transfer to a large bowl.
7. Pour lemon juice mixture over pasta; toss to coat well.
8. Add ricotta cheese and toss; add cooked vegetables and dill.
9. Toss to mix well.
10. Taste and add more pepper if desired.
11. Garnish with julienned lemon rind.

Variation
Cut 2 oz (50 g) thinly sliced smoked salmon into strips. Toss with pasta mixture.

Makes 2 to 3 servings

1 Serving:
Protein 10 grams
Fat 10 grams
Carbohydrate 45 grams
Calories 310

Lentil Salad with Roasted Red Peppers

Quick and easy using canned legumes and roasted peppers, this salad provides a perfect protein complement with our multi-grain bread or couscous.

1	19 oz (540 mL) can lentils, drained OR 2 cups (500 mL) cooked dried lentils	1
¾ cup	chopped, canned roasted sweet red peppers	175 mL
¼ cup	sliced green onions	50 mL
3 tbsp.	lemon juice	50 mL
2 tbsp.	olive oil	25 mL
2	cloves garlic, finely minced	2
½ tsp.	dried basil	2 mL
½ tsp.	dried thyme	2 mL
½ tsp.	dried oregano	2 mL
	freshly ground pepper	

Optional additions:

½ cup	fresh mint	125 mL
½ bunch	arugula, chopped	½ bunch
4 oz	feta cheese	125 g
	cherry tomatoes	

Makes 4 to 6 servings

1 Serving:
Protein 6 grams
Fat 4 grams
Carbohydrate 17 grams
Calories 128

Method
1. Rinse lentils under cold running water; drain well.
2. In a medium bowl, combine lentils, peppers and onions.
3. In a separate bowl, combine lemon juice, oil, garlic, basil, thyme, oregano and pepper to taste.
4. Stir into lentils.
5. Refrigerate for 2 hours or overnight.

To cook 1 cup (250 mL) of lentils: In heavy saucepan, cover rinsed lentils with 2 cups (500 mL) cold water; bring to a boil, reduce heat and simmer covered until tender (10 to 15 minutes for red lentils, 30 to 45 minutes for green lentils). Drain if necessary. Makes 2 cups (500 mL).

A favorite legume of ours, lentils look like tiny brown or red buttons. Combined with rice, they make a high-protein, stick-to-the-ribs meal.

Brown Rice Salad

½ cup	brown rice	125 mL
1¼ cups	water	300 mL
⅓ cup	Light Vinaigrette (page 111)	75 mL
2 tbsp.	lemon juice	25 mL
¼ tsp.	dried basil	1 mL
¼ tsp.	dried oregano	1 mL
1 to 2	cloves garlic, minced	1 to 2
	freshly ground pepper	
1	tomato, diced	1
1½ cup	coarsely chopped sweet red or green peppers	125 mL
½ cup	coarsely chopped zucchini	125 mL
2 tbsp.	minced fresh parsley	25 mL
2 tbsp.	finely chopped red or Spanish onion	25 mL
¼ cup	diced part-skim mozzarella cheese (optional)	50 mL

Method

1. In a 3 qt. (3 L) microwaveable container combine rice and water.
2. Cover and microwave at High for 3 to 6 minutes or until boiling.
3. **Microwave at Medium (50%)** for 15 to 17 minutes or until most of liquid is absorbed and rice is tender; let stand for 5 to 10 minutes. OR **cook on top of stove** for about 30 to 40 minutes.
4. In a small bowl, mix together vinaigrette, lemon juice, basil, oregano, garlic and pepper to taste.
5. Stir into rice; add tomato, peppers, zucchini, parsley and onion.
6. Refrigerate for at least 1 hour or overnight.
7. Just before serving stir in cheese if using.

Brown rice is an excellent source of B vitamins. Let the microwave shorten the cooking time for this delicious fresh-tasting salad.

Makes 4 side salads or 2 main course servings

1 Side Salad:
Protein 2 grams
Fat 5 grams
Carbohydrate 23 grams
Calories 145

Brown rice is white rice with the outer hull removed but the bran layer left on, making it the most nutritious rice and higher in fiber. It has a somewhat nutty flavor and chewy texture when cooked.

Wild Rice and Orange Salad

Serve as part of an "uptown" buffet after an afternoon match. Entertain guests with this elegant, fresh-tasting salad and complete with grilled chicken for a gathering easy on the host or hostess.

½ cup	wild rice, rinsed	125 mL
2 cups	chicken stock	500 mL
¼ cup	orange juice	50 mL
1 tbsp.	olive oil	15 mL
2 tsp.	grated orange rind	10 mL
⅛ tsp.	ground ginger	0.5 mL
⅛ tsp.	ground cinnamon	0.5 mL
	freshly ground pepper	
2	oranges, peeled and sectioned (about 1 cup/250 mL)	2
¼ cup	raisins	50 mL
2 tbsp.	chopped fresh mint	25 mL
	mint sprigs for garnish	

Makes 3 servings

1 Serving:
Protein 3.5 grams
Fat 4.5 grams
Carbohydrate 49 grams
Calories 250

Method

1. In a medium saucepan, combine rice and stock; cover and bring to boil.
2. Reduce heat and simmer for 45 to 50 minutes or until rice is tender; drain off excess liquid.
3. Mix together orange juice, oil, rind, ginger, cinnamon and pepper to taste; pour over warm rice.
4. Add orange segments, raisins and mint.
5. Cover and refrigerate for 2 hours or overnight.
6. Garnish with mint sprigs.

Wild rice is not really a rice but is the seed of aquatic grass. It has a delicious nutty flavor, a chewy texture and it makes an interesting addition to rice pilaf.

Wehani is an aromatic gourmet American brown rice and is longer grained than regular long-grain brown rice. It is rust in color and smells like corn popping when cooking. It is more expensive, so used on special occasions.

Middle Eastern Chickpea Salad

1	19 oz (540 mL) can chickpeas, drained and rinsed	1
1 cup	seeded and diced tomato	250 mL
½ cup	chopped fresh parsley	125 mL
2 tbsp.	chopped red or Spanish onion	25 mL
⅔ cup	Light Vinaigrette (page 111)	150 mL
2	cloves garlic, minced	2
½ tsp.	ground cumin	2 mL
½ tsp.	ground coriander (cilantro)	2 mL

Method

1. In a medium bowl, combine chickpeas, tomato, parsley and onion.
2. Mix vinaigrette, garlic, cumin and coriander.
3. Pour over chickpea mixture; stir to combine.
4. Cover and refrigerate for at least 1 hour or overnight.

Variation

Add grilled chicken for a more substantial meal.

The flavors in this dressing complement each other in the best Middle Eastern tradition. Chickpeas are an excellent alternate protein source and are high in fiber.

Makes 3 to 4 servings

1 Serving:
Protein 9 grams
Fat 12 grams
Carbohydrate 28 grams
Calories 256

Garbanzos in Spanish, ceci in Italian, chickpeas are round and beige. Widely used in Mediterranean countries in soups, salads and spreads, these are a low-budget high-protein boon to menus.

Skiing was used by the Swedes as a military technique in warfare in the Middle Ages before spreading to other countries. Skiing did not become an organized sport until the last half of the 19th century and is now Norway's national sport.

Southwest Black Bean Salad

The earthy, distinctive flavor of these legumes is hotly sparked by jalapeno peppers and fresh coriander. The lively taste of this salad belies its healthy goodness.

½ cup	dried black beans	125 mL
½ cup	chopped sweet green or yellow pepper	125 mL
½ cup	frozen corn niblets, thawed OR cooked fresh corn niblets	125 mL
¼ cup	chopped red or Spanish onion	50 mL
3 tbsp.	white vinegar	50 mL
2 tbsp.	chopped fresh coriander (cilantro)	25 mL
1 tbsp.	olive oil	15 mL
2 to 3 tsp.	chopped jalapeno peppers or canned green chilies	10 to 15 mL
¼ tsp.	salt	1 mL

Makes 4 to 5 servings

1 Serving:
Protein 5 grams
Fat 3 grams
Carbohydrate 17 grams
Calories 115

Method

1. Rinse the beans; place in saucepan and add 1½ cups (375 mL) cold water.
2. Cover and bring to boil; boil for 3 minutes.
3. Remove from heat and let soak for 20 minutes; drain.
4. In the same pan, combine beans and 1½ cups (375 mL) cold water; cover and bring to boil; simmer for 1 hour or just until tender. Drain.
5. In bowl, combine beans, green pepper, corn and onion.
6. Mix together vinegar, coriander, oil, jalapeno peppers and salt.
7. Pour over bean mixture; stir to combine.
8. Marinate in refrigerator for at least 2 hours or up to 24 hours.

French Potato Salad

2	large new red or white potatoes	2
2 tbsp.	minced fresh parsley	25 mL
1 tbsp.	white wine vinegar	15 mL
1 tbsp.	olive oil	15 mL
1 tsp.	Dijon mustard	5 mL
1	shallot, minced	1
¼ tsp.	salt	1 mL
¼ tsp.	freshly ground pepper	1 mL

Microwave Method

1. Scrub potatoes and cut into large bite-sized pieces.
2. In a 4 cup (1 L) microwaveable casserole, combine potatoes with 2 tbsp (25 mL) water.
3. Cover and microwave at High for 6 to 7 minutes, or just until tender, stirring once; drain well.
4. Mix parsley, vinegar, oil, mustard, shallots, salt and pepper; pour over warm potatoes.
5. Toss gently to coat.
6. Allow to marinate for 1 to 2 hours at room temperature or refrigerate overnight.

Creamy Variation

Add 2 tbsp. (25 mL) low fat yogurt and ½ tsp. (2 mL) dried tarragon to parsley mixture in step 4.

Variation

Potato Salad Nicoise: Add ½ tsp. oregano, 1 clove of garlic crushed and 1 lb (500 g) of green beans, steamed, to step 4.

Potato salad doesn't have to be "heavy on the mayo" to be delicious. Serve this recipe with grilled hamburgers as a hearty reward for a marathon jog.

Makes 2 to 3 servings

1 Serving:
Protein 2.5 grams
Fat 4.5 grams
Carbohydrate 21 grams
Calories 135

Warm Szechuan Chicken Salad

A stir-fry that's really a salad, this hot and spicy recipe makes a satisfying weekend lunch or weeknight supper.

3 cups	salad greens	750 mL
¼ cup	Light Vinaigrette (page 111)	50 mL
1 tsp.	soy sauce	5 mL
½ tsp.	finely minced fresh gingerroot	2 mL
⅛ to ¼ tsp.	crushed chili peppers	0.5 to 1 mL
2 tsp.	vegetable oil	10 mL
4 oz	boneless, skinless chicken breast, thinly sliced	125 g
8	snow peas, cut into bite-sized pieces	8
2	green onions, sliced	2
2 tbsp.	diced sweet red or yellow pepper	25 mL
2 tbsp.	unsalted peanuts for garnish	25 mL

Method

1. Tear salad greens into a salad bowl.
2. Mix vinaigrette, soy sauce, ginger and chili peppers; set aside.
3. In a small non-stick skillet, heat oil over medium-high heat. Add chicken and stir-fry for about 2 minutes until no longer pink inside.
4. Add snow peas, green onion and red pepper; stir-fry for 1 minute.
5. Add vinaigrette mixture and simmer for 1 to 2 minutes or until vegetables are tender-crisp.
6. Spoon over greens; toss.
7. Garnish with peanuts, if using, and serve immediately.

Scallop Variation
For seafood lovers, substitute cooked scallops for chicken.

Makes 2 servings

1 Serving:
Protein 18 grams
Fat 14 grams
Carbohydrate 11 grams
Calories 242

Santa Fe-Style Warm Salad

3 cups	salad greens	750 mL
¼ cup	Light Vinaigrette (page 111)	50 mL
2 tsp.	lime juice	10 mL
⅛ to ¼ tsp.	crushed dried chilies	0.5 to 1 mL
2 tsp.	vegetable oil	10 mL
4 oz	beef sirloin, thinly sliced	125 g
8	snow peas, trimmed and cut in bite-sized pieces	8
2	green onions, sliced	2
2 tbsp.	diced sweet red or yellow pepper	25 mL
2 tbsp.	minced fresh coriander (cilantro)	25 mL

Method

1. Tear salad greens into salad bowl.
2. Mix vinaigrette, lime juice and chilies; set aside.
3. In a non-stick skillet, heat oil over medium-high heat; add beef and stir-fry for about 2 minutes or until browned but still pink inside.
4. Transfer to bowl of salad greens.
5. To skillet, add snow peas, green onions and red pepper; stir-fry for 1 minute.
6. Add vinaigrette mixture and simmer for 1 minute or until vegetables are tender-crisp.
7. Spoon over greens; toss.
8. Sprinkle with coriander and serve immediately.

Fresh coriander and chilies give a warm Southwestern flavor to this main dish salad. Tasty and colorful, this recipe is special enough to treat the athlete you love.

Makes 2 servings

1 Serving:
Protein 18 grams
Fat 11 grams
Carbohydrate 11 grams
Calories 215

Early skis or wooden "gliding shoes" up to twelve feet long were used by Scandinavian gold prospectors in 1849 as a means of travel as well as for downhill racing competitions.

Marinated Bean Salad

A lighter updated version of everyone's old family favorite. Still a great dish for reunions, with the nutritious bonus of protein, fiber and complex carbohydrate.

2 cups	cooked green beans	500 mL
1	19 oz (540 mL) can white kidney beans, drained and rinsed	1
1	19 oz (540 mL) can red kidney beans, drained and rinsed	1
1	19 oz (540 mL) can chickpeas, drained and rinsed	1
¾ cup	sliced Vidalia, Spanish or red onion	175 mL
½ cup	chopped sweet green pepper	125 mL
½ cup	chopped sweet red pepper or pimento	125 mL
½ cup	chopped fresh parsley	125 mL
1 cup	chicken stock	250 mL
⅓ cup	cider vinegar	75 mL
¼ cup	vegetable oil	50 mL
4	cloves garlic, minced	4
2 tsp.	honey	10 mL
1 tsp.	dried oregano	5 mL
1 tsp.	dried thyme	5 mL
1 tsp.	freshly ground pepper	5 mL

Makes 8 cups (2 L)

1 Cup:
Protein 13 grams
Fat 7 grams
Carbohydrate 40 grams
Calories 275

Method

1. In a large bowl, combine green beans, white and red kidney beans, chickpeas, onion, green pepper, red pepper and parsley.
2. In a small bowl, mix chicken stock, vinegar, oil, garlic, honey, oregano, thyme and pepper; pour over bean mixture.
3. Stir to coat well.
4. Marinate in refrigerator for 4 hours or up to 4 days, stirring occasionally.

▦　　▦　　▦　　▦　　▦　　▦　　▦

Summer Holiday Picnic

Marinated Bean Salad

Rosemary Grilled Chicken (page 198)

Brown Rice Salad (page 119)

Almond Brownie Bites (page 237)

Fresh Berries

Allan's Marinated Tomato Salad

2	large tomatoes, cored and cut in wedges	2
½ cup	sliced Spanish onion	125 mL
1 tbsp.	olive oil	15 mL
¼ cup	fresh basil leaves	50 mL
	freshly ground pepper	
⅓ cup	diced feta cheese	75 mL

Method
1. In a medium bowl, combine tomato, onion and oil.
2. If basil leaves are large, tear into smaller pieces; add to tomatoes.
3. Toss and season with pepper to taste.
4. Marinate at room temperature for 30 minutes.
5. Add cheese; toss and serve.

This salad, bursting with vitamin C and lycopene, is at its juicy best with summer-ripe beefsteak tomatoes. Serve with thick slices of crusty bread or use as a "no cook" pasta sauce.

Makes 2 servings

1 Serving:
Protein 8 grams
Fat 16 grams
Carbohydrate 14 grams
Calories 232

Greek-Style Leeks Vinaigrette

The "poor man's asparagus," leeks topped with feta cheese make a full-bodied appetizer or side salad. Serve with a glass of retsina and hunks of crusty bread.

2	leeks	2
¾ cup	hot water	175 mL
¼ tsp.	chicken stock granules	1 mL
2 tbsp.	tarragon vinegar*	25 mL
1 tbsp.	olive oil	15 mL
½ tsp.	Dijon mustard	2 mL
1	small clove garlic, minced	1
	freshly ground black pepper	
2 to 4	Boston, Bibb or romaine lettuce leaves	2 to 4
2 tbsp.	crumbled feta cheese (about 1 oz/30 g)	25 mL
1 tbsp.	chopped fresh parsley	15 mL
1 tbsp.	diced red pepper or pimento	15 mL

*If not available, substitute 2 tbsp. (25 mL) white wine vinegar and ¼ tsp. (1 mL) dried tarragon.

Makes 2 servings

1 Serving:
Protein 3 grams
Fat 10 grams
Carbohydrate 4 grams
Calories 118

Method

1. Trim off woody green end of leeks; slit leeks lengthwise leaving bulb intact.
2. Wash carefully to remove grit.
3. Place in a skillet or saucepan; mix water and chicken stock granules and pour over leeks.
4. Cover and bring to boil; reduce heat and simmer until leeks are tender, about 10 to 15 minutes.
5. Reserve 1 tbsp. (15 mL) liquid; then drain.
6. Meanwhile, combine vinegar, oil, reserved liquid, mustard, garlic and pepper to taste; mix well.
7. Pour over warm leeks; marinate for 2 to 3 hours at room temperature or refrigerate for 1 to 2 days.
8. To serve, arrange leeks on lettuce leaves and sprinkle cheese, parsley and red pepper over top.

Variation

Substitute ½ lb (250 g) fresh asparagus for leeks, adjusting cooking time as necessary.

Watercress and Beets Vinaigrette (page 116)
Zucchini Frittata (page 138)

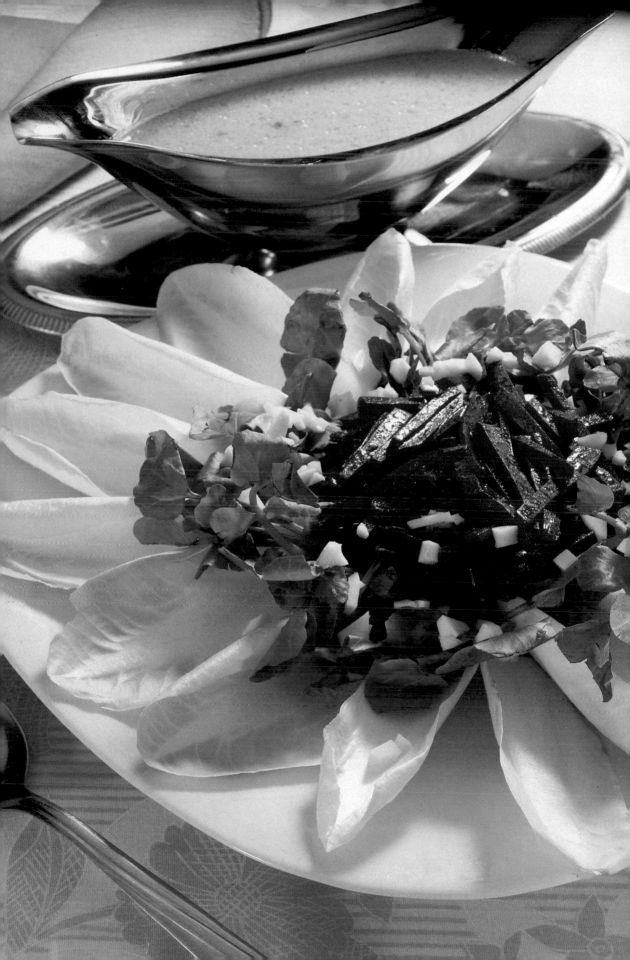

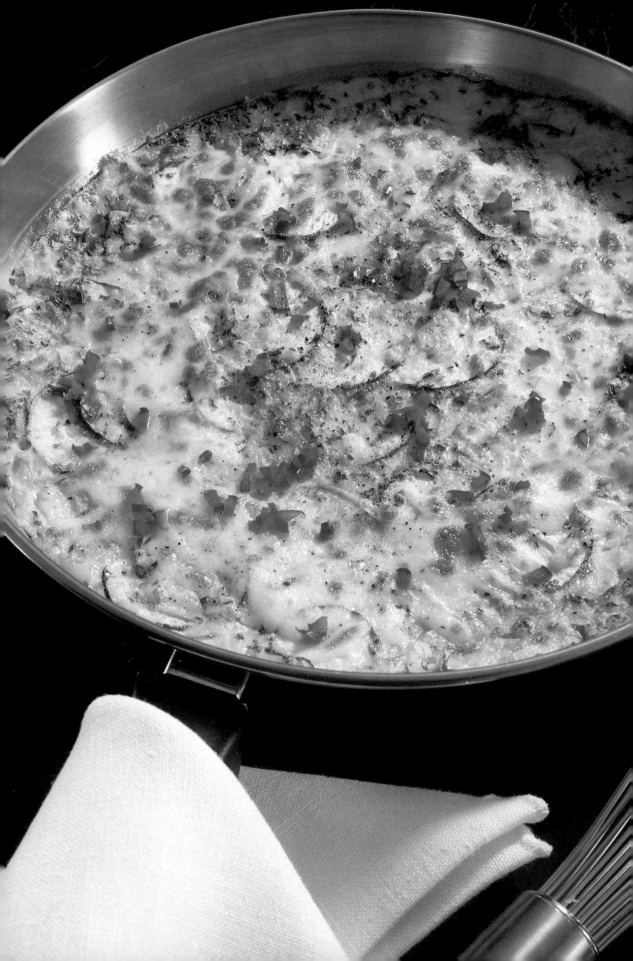

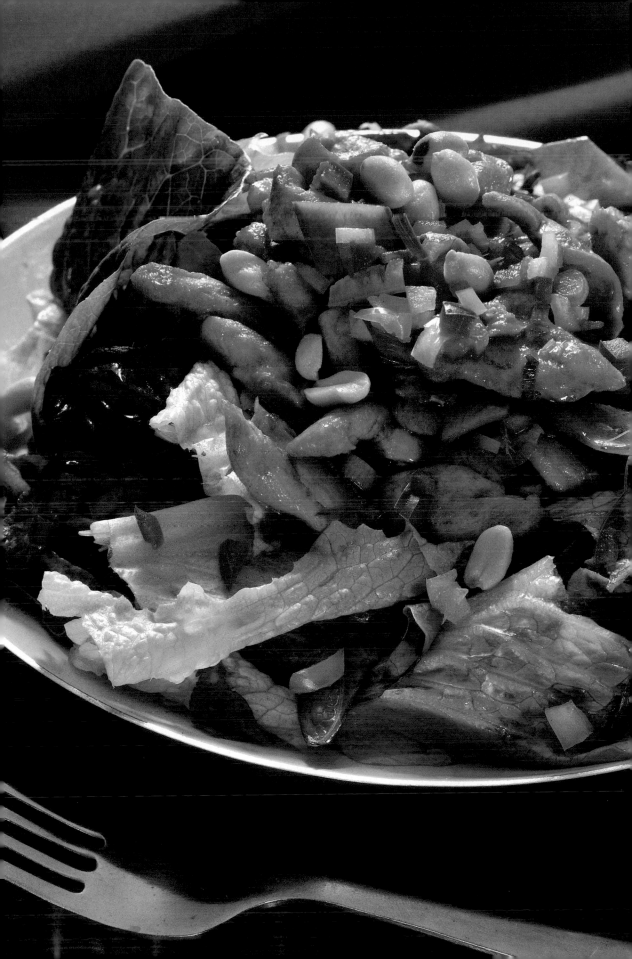

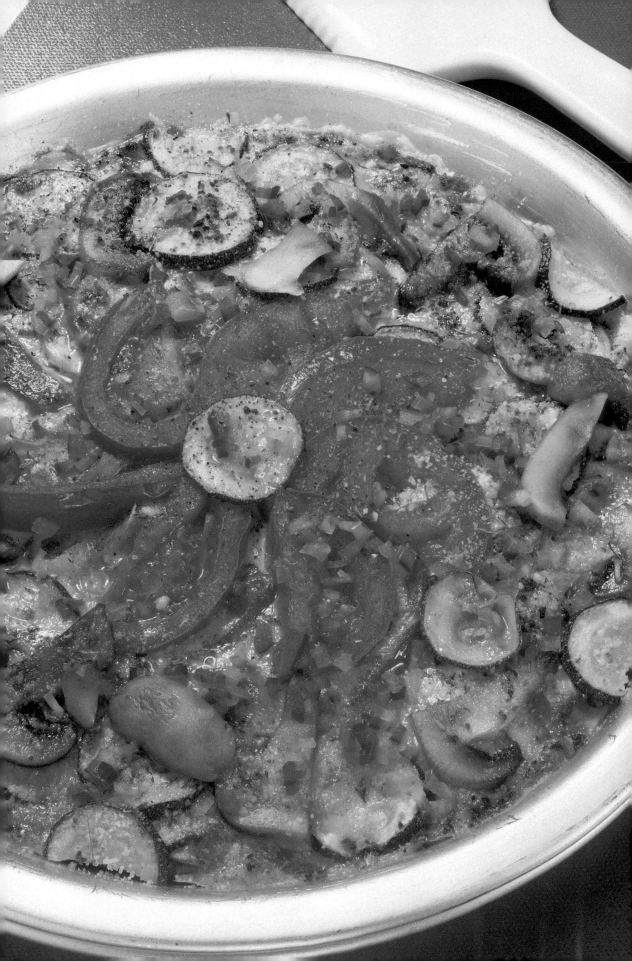

Technicolor Coleslaw

3 cups	finely shredded green cabbage	750 mL
1 cup	grated carrots	250 mL
1 cup	julienned sweet red or green peppers	250 mL
2	green onions, sliced	2
¼ cup	2% plain yogurt	50 mL
2 tbsp	light mayonnaise	25 mL
2 tsp.	Dijon mustard	10 mL
1 tsp.	2% milk	5 mL
½ tsp.	granulated sugar	2 mL
¼ tsp.	caraway or celery seeds	1 mL
¼ tsp.	freshly ground pepper	1 mL
	unsalted peanuts for garnish	

Adapted from a family recipe, enjoy this salad as is, or with our Light Vinaigrette (page 111) for a tart and refreshing change. Cabbage is one of the brassica vegetables which may help reduce the risk of colon cancer.

Method

1. In a large bowl, combine cabbage, carrots, peppers and green onions.
2. In another bowl, combine yogurt, mayonnaise, mustard, milk, sugar, seeds and pepper; mix well.
3. Pour over cabbage mixture; toss well.
4. Garnish with peanuts.

Makes 4 servings

1 Serving:
Protein 1 gram
Fat 3 grams
Carbohydrate 8 grams
Calories 63

Warm Szechuan Chicken Salad (page 124)
Fast Lane Pizza (page 134)

Apple and Pepper Squash Salad

This salad with its contrast of crisp apples and mellow squash is a unique combination of fall fruits and vegetables.

2 tbsp.	chopped leek (white part only)	25 mL
2 tbsp.	dry white wine	25 mL
1 tbsp.	red wine vinegar	15 mL
1 tbsp.	chicken stock	15 mL
¼ tsp.	dry mustard	1 mL
¼ tsp.	salt	1 mL
⅛ tsp.	granulated sugar	0.5 mL
pinch	freshly ground pepper	pinch
2 tbsp.	olive oil	25 mL
1	pepper or butternut squash (1¼ lb/550 g)	1
1	medium McIntosh apple	1
1 tbsp.	finely chopped red onion	15 mL
	lettuce leaves	
2 tbsp.	toasted walnut halves for garnish	15 mL

Method

1. In a small saucepan, combine leeks and wine; cook over medium heat, stirring often, 2 to 3 minutes or until wine has evaporated. Let cool.
2. In a small bowl, combine vinegar, chicken stock, mustard, salt, sugar and pepper. Gradually whisk in oil. Add leeks and set aside.
3. Cut squash in half, scoop out seeds and peel.
4. Cut into ½ inch (1 cm) cubes.
5. Cook squash in boiling water just until tender but not mushy, 5 to 8 minutes.
6. Drain and cool under cold running water.
7. Drain and arrange on paper towels to absorb excess moisture.
8. Core apple leaving skin on and cut into ½ inch (1 cm) cubes.
9. Combine squash, apple, onion and leek mixture. Chill for 30 minutes.
10. Taste and adjust seasoning with pepper.
11. Spoon salad onto lettuce leaves.
12. Garnish with walnuts.

Makes 4 servings

1 Serving:
Protein 2 grams
Fat 9 grams
Carbohydrate 19 grams
Calories 165

Tip

To toast walnuts: Spread walnuts on a pie plate or baking sheet; bake in 350°F (180°C) oven for 10 to 15 minutes or until fragrant.

To soften squash for easy cutting: Pierce squash all over; microwave at High for 2 to 3 minutes.

Oriental Slaw

2 cups	shredded red cabbage	500 mL
½ cup	thinly sliced celery	125 mL
⅓ cup	thinly sliced red or Spanish onion	75 mL
2 tbsp.	rice or cider vinegar	25 mL
1 tbsp.	vegetable oil	15 mL
1 tbsp.	honey	15 mL
1	small clove garlic, minced	1
1 tsp.	minced fresh gingerroot	5 mL
¼ tsp.	freshly ground pepper	1 mL
⅛ tsp.	salt	0.5 mL
2 tsp.	toasted sesame seeds	10 mL

Crisp in texture, this slaw has a delicate, slightly sweet dressing. Serve this with lean grilled pork as an excellent way to get the brassica group into your diet.

Method

1. In a medium bowl, combine cabbage, celery and onion.
2. In a 1 cup (250 mL) measure, combine vinegar, oil, honey, garlic, ginger, pepper and salt.
3. **Microwave** uncovered at High for 1 minute or until heated through and stir. OR **heat in saucepan** over medium heat.
4. Pour over vegetables; toss to mix well.
5. Sprinkle sesame seeds on top.
6. Serve immediately.

Makes 2 to 3 servings

1 Serving:
Protein 1.5 grams
Fat 6 grams
Carbohydrate 11 grams
Calories 104

Tip
To toast sesame seeds: In small skillet, cook seeds over medium heat for about 5 minutes or until golden, shaking often.

Eggs, Cheese and Pizza:
egg-stracting power to spare

Calzone

This tasty pizza has the usual toppings tucked inside a pocket of crispy crust. Eat out of hand at home for a casual meal after weight training or low impact aerobics.

1½ tsp.	olive oil	7 mL
½ cup	sliced mushrooms	125 mL
¼ cup	diced sweet green or red pepper	50 mL
8 oz	fresh OR frozen and thawed whole wheat or white pizza dough or bread dough	250 g
¼ cup	2% cottage cheese	50 mL
1 tbsp.	grated Parmesan cheese	15 mL
1 tbsp.	chopped fresh basil OR 1 tsp.(5 mL) dried	15 mL
½ tsp.	fennel or anise seeds	2 mL
⅓ cup	Basic Tomato Sauce (page 214) OR canned pizza sauce	75 mL
½ tsp.	cornmeal	2 mL

Makes 2 servings

1 Serving:
Protein 13 grams
Fat 4 grams
Carbohydrate 62 grams
Calories 336

Method

1. In a non–stick skillet, heat 1 tsp. (5 mL) oil over medium-high heat; cook mushrooms and peppers for 3 to 5 minutes or until tender. Let cool.
2. Cut dough into 2 equal pieces; roll into circles.
3. Set aside to rest for 10 minutes and then roll again to a 7 inch (17 cm) diameter.
4. In a small bowl, mix cottage cheese, 1 tbsp. (15 mL) Parmesan cheese, basil and fennel seeds together.
5. Divide cheese mixture over one-half of each circle of dough leaving a ½ inch (1 cm) border around the outside.
6. Arrange peppers and mushrooms on top of cheese.
7. Spoon tomato sauce evenly over vegetables (if using Basic Tomato Sauce, drain in a sieve).
8. Moisten edges lightly with water.
9. Fold other side of circle over filling and press 2 edges together firmly with fingers to seal.
10. Brush surface lightly with remaining olive oil.
11. Sprinkle cornmeal on top.
12. Bake in lower half of 425°F (220°C) oven for 12 to 15 minutes or until crisp and brown.
13. Let stand for 5 minutes before serving.

Fennel or anise seeds resemble licorice in flavor and produce a taste that is distinctly Italian.

Artichoke Pizza

8 oz	fresh OR frozen and thawed whole wheat or white pizza dough or bread dough	250 g
1 tbsp.	cornmeal	15 mL
¾ cup	Basic Tomato Sauce (page 214) OR canned pizza sauce	175 mL
1 tbsp.	chopped fresh basil OR 1 tsp. (5 mL) dried	15 mL
1 tbsp.	grated Parmesan cheese	15 mL
1 cup	sliced fresh mushrooms	250 mL
¾ cup	canned artichoke hearts, drained and cut in eighths (about 2 artichoke hearts)	175 mL
½ cup	thinly sliced sweet red, green or yellow pepper	125 mL
½ cup	diced lean cooked ham (about 2 oz/60 g)	125 mL
1 cup	grated part-skim mozzarella cheese	250 mL

Method

1. Roll or stretch dough into a 10 inch (25 cm) circle.
2. Sprinkle baking sheet or pizza pan with cornmeal.
3. Place dough on pan; cover with plastic wrap and let rise for 30 minutes.
4. Meanwhile, prepare topping ingredients. If using Basic Tomato Sauce, drain in a sieve. In a small bowl, mix tomato sauce, basil and Parmesan cheese. Spread on crust, leaving ½ inch (1 cm) border around the outside.
5. Arrange mushrooms, artichoke hearts, peppers and ham on top of sauce.
6. Sprinkle mozzarella cheese over top.
7. Bake in lower half of 475°F (240°C) oven for 12 to 18 minutes or until bottom is crisp and browned.
8. Cut in wedges to serve.

Preparation time is reduced dramatically using fresh or frozen bread dough. The fresh vegetables and lean ham make a complete meal when topped with Parmesan cheese.

Makes 2 to 4 servings

1 Serving:
Protein 18 grams
Fat 6 grams
Carbohydrate 37 grams
Calories 274

The artichoke is a low calorie vegetable that has been a delicacy in Europe for 400 years. Canned artichoke hearts can be high in sodium.

Fast Lane Pizza

Pita bread makes an equally good pizza crust when time is of the essence. This short cut is delicious and fresh tasting.

2 tbsp.	olive oil	25 mL
1 cup	sliced onion	250 mL
1	large clove garlic, minced	1
1½ cups	sliced zucchini	375 mL
1½ cups	sliced mushrooms	375 mL
½ cup	diced sweet green pepper	125 mL
1	6 in. (16 cm) whole wheat pita	1
2	fresh tomatoes, sliced	2
1 tbsp.	chopped fresh basil OR	15 mL
	1 tsp. (5 mL) dried	
1 tbsp.	chopped fresh oregano OR	15 mL
	1 tsp. (5 mL) dried	
	freshly ground pepper	
1½ cups	grated part-skim mozzarella cheese	375 mL
2 tbsp.	grated Parmesan cheese	25 mL

Makes 4 to 5 servings

1 Serving:
Protein 16 grams
Fat 12 grams
Carbohydrate 33 grams
Calories 304

Method

1. In a large non-stick skillet, heat oil over medium high-heat. Add onions and garlic; sauté for 2 to 3 minutes or until onions are softened.
2. Add zucchini, mushrooms, green pepper and sauté for 3 to 4 minutes or until vegetables are tender.
3. Split pita breads horizontally by cutting around the outside edge with scissors. Overlap pita rounds in a 9 inch (22 cm) pie plate.
4. Spoon sautéed vegetable mixture on pita crust.
5. Top with sliced tomatoes; sprinkle with basil, oregano and pepper to taste.
6. Top with mozzarella and Parmesan cheese.
7. Bake in 375°F (190°C) oven for 10 to 15 minutes or until cheese has melted and pitas are crisp.

Popeye's Casserole

1	10 oz (284 g) bag fresh spinach	1	
½ cup	2% cottage cheese	125 mL	
1	egg	1	
1 tbsp.	chopped fresh dill OR 1 tsp. (5 mL) dried	15 mL	
⅛ tsp.	ground nutmeg freshly ground pepper	0.5 mL	
¼ cup	grated old Cheddar cheese	50 mL	
2 tbsp.	unsalted sunflower seeds	25 mL	

That old salt got his power from spinach. You will too, with this main course that is rich in vitamins, minerals and protein, yet low in calories.

Method

1. Wash spinach and remove coarse stems.
2. In a small amount of boiling water, **steam** spinach just until wilted. OR **microwave** covered at High for about 3 minutes.
3. Drain very well, squeezing out excess moisture; chop finely.
4. Add cottage cheese, egg, dill, nutmeg and pepper to taste.
5. Spoon spinach mixture into lightly greased 1 qt. (1 L) casserole.
6. Sprinkle Cheddar cheese and sunflower seeds on top.
7. Bake in 350°F (180°C) oven for 20 to 30 minutes or until set in the center.

Makes 2 to 3 servings

1 Serving:
Protein 14 grams
Fat 7.5 grams
Carbohydrate 6 grams
Calories 148

Sunflower seeds, with approximately 25 per cent protein and just under 50 per cent fat by weight, are almost 20 per cent protein as a percentage of total calories. Seeds add texture, variety and nutritional balance to meals and shouldn't be relegated to just a snack.

Comfort Supper

This baked potato is a meal in itself and comforting in its cheesy heartiness. Simple to make and great for a casual supper.

2	large baking potatoes	2
1 cup	Indispensable Cheese Sauce (page 215) made with Cheddar cheese, divided	250 mL
1	green onion, sliced	1
¼ tsp.	salt	2 mL
¼ tsp	freshly ground pepper	2 mL
¼ cup	diced cooked beef, ham, chicken or turkey	50 mL
½ cup	cooked vegetables or frozen mixed vegetables, thawed and diced	125 mL

Makes 2 servings

1 Serving:
Protein 21 grams
Fat 12 grams
Carbohydrate 49 grams
Calories 388

Microwave Method

1. Scrub potatoes and prick with fork.
2. Arrange on paper towels in microwave oven and microwave at High for 6 to 8 minutes or until soft when squeezed.
3. Wrap in foil and let stand for 5 minutes; unwrap and cool for 5 minutes.
4. Cut a slice from top of each potato; using a teaspoon, scoop out potato being careful not to break the outer skin.
5. Mash the potato with ¼ cup (50 mL) of Indispensable Cheese Sauce.
6. Mix in green onion, salt, pepper and meat of your choice; spoon back into potato skins.
7. Microwave at High for 2 to 2½ minutes or until heated through.
8. Microwave remaining sauce at Medium (50%) for 1 to 2 minutes or until hot.
9. Stir in vegetables; microwave at High for 30 to 60 seconds or until vegetables are hot.
10. Spoon over each potato.

Variations

Vegetarian Version: Mix 2 tbsp. (25 mL) of sauce with cooked potato, substitute ¼ cup (50 mL) cottage cheese for meat and add ⅛ tsp. (0.5 mL) ground nutmeg.

Simpler Variation: Omit cutting tops off and scooping potato out of skin. Combine all the sauce, vegetables and meat; heat as directed in recipe until hot. Slash the top of each baked potato in a cross; squeeze to open. Spoon sauce over potatoes.

Vegetarian Red Pepper Strata

1 tbsp.	vegetable oil	15 mL
1	red pepper, thinly sliced	1
2	cloves garlic, minced	2
1	leek, sliced (white part only)	1
1 cup	sliced mushrooms	250 mL
10	slices whole grain bread, stale or day-old, cut into 1 inch (2.5 cm) squares	10
1½ cups	grated Cheddar cheese	375 mL
2 cups	milk	500 mL
3	large eggs	3
1 tbsp.	Dijon mustard	15 mL
1 tsp.	basil or oregano	5 mL
1 tsp.	salt	5 mL
½ tsp.	pepper	2 mL
½ cup	parsley, chopped	125 mL

Method

1. Preheat oven to 350°F (180°C). Heat oil in a large skillet over medium-high heat. Add garlic, pepper, leeks and mushrooms. Sauté, stirring, until soft, about 5 minutes. Remove from heat.
2. Scatter half of bread in an 8-inch-square baking dish. Cover with half of the cheese, then half of the pepper mixture. Repeat layering with bread, cheese and pepper mixture.
3. Beat milk, eggs, mustard, basil, salt and pepper in a bowl. Pour over strata. Chill strata, covered, at least 30 minutes and up to 12 hours.
4. Bake until lightly browned on top and set in center, about 45 minutes. Let stand 10 minutes before serving. Garnish with parsley.

This is one of our favorites for fall-out-of-bed entertaining in the a.m. Updated to reduce the fat and packed with colorful, tasty vegetables, this entrée will have guests begging for seconds! Make the night before to have a stress-free brunch.

4 to 6 servings

1 Serving:
Protein 19 grams
Fat 15 grams
Carbohydrate 34 grams
Calories 347

Zucchini Frittata

An Italian-style omelet, this entrée began its history as humble peasant food. We recommend that like the workers in centuries past, you pack any leftovers in a sandwich for lunch.

1 tbsp.	olive oil	15 mL
½ cup	chopped sweet red, yellow or orange pepper	125 mL
⅓ cup	chopped onion	75 mL
1½ cups	sliced zucchini	375 mL
4	eggs	4
2	egg whites	2
¼ cup	2% milk	50 mL
¼ cup	grated Parmesan cheese	50 mL
2 tsp.	dried basil OR 2 tbsp. (25 mL) fresh	10 mL
⅛ tsp.	salt	0.5 mL
	freshly ground pepper	
½ cup	grated part-skim mozzarella cheese (optional)	125 mL

Method

1. In a medium non-stick skillet, heat oil over medium-high heat. Add red pepper and onion; sauté for 2 to 3 minutes or until softened.
2. Add zucchini and sauté for 3 to 4 minutes or until partially cooked.
3. In a medium bowl beat eggs, egg whites, milk, Parmesan cheese, basil, salt and pepper. Pour over vegetables in skillet.
4. Cook over medium heat lifting outer edges to allow uncooked egg to run to the bottom.
5. Cover and cook until set but still moist on the surface.
6. Sprinkle with mozzarella cheese if using. Let stand covered for 5 minutes to melt cheese or place under broiler for 2 to 3 minutes to brown lightly. (If handle of skillet isn't oven-proof, wrap with foil.)
7. Cut in wedges and serve hot or at room temperature.

Makes 6 servings
Protein 10 grams
Fat 10 grams
Carbohydrate 3 grams
Calories 142

Tip
When making egg dishes, you can reduce fat and cholesterol by increasing the proportion of whites to egg yolks.

Pissaladière

8 oz	fresh OR frozen and thawed whole wheat or white pizza dough or bread dough	250 g
2 tbsp.	olive oil	25 mL
3 cups	sliced onions, separated into rings	750 mL
⅓ cup	diced sweet red pepper	75 mL
1 tsp	dried oregano OR 1 tbsp. (15 mL) fresh	5 mL
	freshly ground pepper	
12	black olives, pitted and sliced	12

Method

1. Roll or stretch dough into a 10 inch (25 cm) circle.
2. Place on a non-stick baking sheet or pizza pan; cover with plastic wrap and let rise for 30 minutes.
3. Meanwhile, in a large non-stick skillet, heat oil over medium heat; add onions and sauté for 7 to 10 minutes or until limp, stirring often.
4. Stir in red pepper and oregano; add pepper to taste. Let cool.
5. Spread onion mixture on dough; sprinkle with black olive slices.
6. Bake in lower half of 400°F (200°C) oven for 20 to 25 minutes or until bottom is crisp and browned.
7. Cut in wedges.
8. Serve warm or at room temperature.

Inspired by Provence, this pizza is topped with sweet, sautéed onions instead of the traditional tomato sauce. Colorful, flavorful, simply wonderful!

Makes 2 to 3 servings

1 Serving:
Protein 7 grams
Fat 11 grams
Carbohydrate 44 grams
Calories 303

Quesadillas

Mexican-style pizza is an easy oven snack spicy enough to take the chill off any skier.

1	10 inch (25 cm) white or whole wheat flour tortilla	1
¼ cup	grated part–skim mozzarella cheese	50 mL
¼ cup	grated medium Cheddar cheese	50 mL
¼ cup	diced green chilies or jalapeno peppers	50 mL
2 tbsp.	Santa Fe Salsa (page 213)	25 mL

Makes 2 lunch servings or 4 snack servings

1 Lunch Serving:
Protein 11 grams
Fat 8 grams
Carbohydrate 29 grams
Calories 232

Method

1. Place tortillas on baking sheet and heat on lowest rack of 375°F (190°C) oven until slightly brown and crisp, about 5 minutes.
2. Sprinkle cheeses and chilies evenly over tortilla.
3. Bake for about 5 minutes or until cheese melts and bottom is crisp.
4. Cut in wedges with pizza cutter or knife.
5. Top each wedge with Santa Fe Salsa.

Variation

Mexican Grilled Cheese Sandwich: Wrap tortillas in foil and **bake** in 350°F (180°C) oven for 5 minutes OR place on paper towels and **microwave** at High for 30 to 45 seconds or just until soft and pliable. Cover one-half of tortilla with cheese and chilies; fold free half of tortilla over cheese and gently press to seal edges. Place on baking sheet and bake in 350°F (180°C) oven for 5 to 10 minutes or until cheese has melted. Serve with 2% plain yogurt and Santa Fe Salsa.

The origins of all sports stem from the time when survival ceased to be the all-consuming preoccupation of humans.

Pesto Pizza

8 oz	fresh OR frozen and thawed whole wheat or white pizza dough or bread dough	250 g
1 tbsp.	cornmeal	15 mL
½ cup	Light Pesto sauce(page 212)	125 mL
1½ cups	coarsely chopped tomatoes OR 14 oz (398 mL) can tomatoes, drained and chopped	375 mL
1 tbsp.	grated Parmesan cheese freshly ground pepper	15 mL
4 oz	creamy goat cheese (chèvre) (about ½ cup/125 mL)	125 g

A pizza to die for! Crisp crust with a fresh pesto topping, this pizza goes for the gold in taste.

Method
1. Roll or stretch dough into 10 inch (25 cm) circle.
2. Sprinkle baking sheet or pizza pan with cornmeal. Place dough on pan; cover with plastic wrap and let rise for 30 minutes.
3. Spread Light Pesto on dough; cover with tomatoes.
4. Sprinkle Parmesan cheese and pepper to taste on tomatoes.
5. Dot pizza with small pieces of goat cheese.
6. Bake in lower half of 475°F (240°C) oven for 12 to 18 minutes or until bottom is crisp.
7. Cut into 8 wedges.

Makes 2 to 4 servings

1 Serving:
Protein 16 grams
Fat 16 grams
Carbohydrate 43 grams
Calories 380

Uptown Saturday Night

Romaine Salad with Light Caesar
   Dressing (page 113)
Pesto Pizza
Fresh Fruit Brûlé (page 232)

Crustless Eggplant Pizza

This is a knife and fork pizza you'll be glad to sink your teeth into. Suitable as an entrée, team with a green salad and fresh fruit for a nicely balanced wholesome meal.

Makes 1 main dish or 2 appetizer servings

1 Serving:
Protein 3 grams
Fat 6 grams
Carbohydrate 6 grams
Calories 90

2	½ inch (1 cm) slices unpeeled eggplant	2
2 tsp.	olive oil	10 mL
2 tbsp.	Basic Tomato Sauce (page 214)	25 mL
2 tbsp.	grated part-skim mozzarella cheese	25 mL
1 tsp.	grated Parmesan cheese	5 mL

Method

1. Brush eggplant slices on both sides with oil; place on baking sheet; spread Basic Tomato Sauce evenly on each slice.
2. Sprinkle with mozzarella and Parmesan cheese.
3. Bake in 425°F (220°C) oven for 10 to 15 minutes or until eggplant is tender and cheese is melted.

Tortilla

2 tsp.	olive oil	10 mL
1	small potato, peeled and finely diced (about ½ cup/125 mL)	1
¼ cup	finely diced onion	50 mL
1	egg	1
1	egg white	1
⅛ tsp	salt	0.5 mL
	freshly ground pepper	

Tortilla is Spanish for omelet. This one is classic in its simplicity – good olive oil, eggs and potatoes.

Method

1. In a small non-stick skillet, heat oil over medium heat. Add potato and onion; sauté for about 5 minutes or until golden brown; cover and cook over low heat until tender, about 5 minutes.
2. In a small bowl, beat egg, egg white, salt and pepper; pour into skillet over potatoes.
3. Cook over medium-high heat, lifting outside edges to allow uncooked portion to flow to the outside and underneath.
4. Cover and cook until set, increasing heat to brown bottom if necessary.
5. Place an inverted plate over the skillet and invert the omelet onto plate.
6. Slide omelet back into pan, browned side up and cook for about 2 to 3 minutes longer or until bottom is golden.
7. Serve hot or let cool to room temperature.

Makes 1 serving

1 Serving:
Protein 11 grams
Fat 15 grams
Carbohydrate 20 grams
Calories 259

French Omelet

Created by the French, this is the perfect "fast food" for a healthy, satisfying meal at home. Fillings can vary with taste or imagination.

2	eggs	2
2	egg whites	2
2 tbsp.	2% milk	25 mL
⅛ tsp.	salt	0.5 mL
	freshly ground pepper	
1 tsp.	butter or soft margarine	5 mL
	filling of your choice	

Makes 1 serving

1 Serving:
Protein 19 grams
Fat 15 grams
Carbohydrate 1 gram
Calories 215

Method

1. In a small bowl, beat eggs, egg whites, milk, salt and pepper to taste.
2. In a small non-stick omelet pan, melt butter over medium-high heat. Pour egg mixture into pan; cook over medium-high heat. Let it set around outside edge. Shaking pan as omelet cooks, lift outside cooked edges and tilt pan to allow uncooked portion to flow underneath.
3. Cover and cook until center is set but moist on top.
4. Spoon filling over center; fold in half and slide onto plate.

Omelet Fillings

1. ¼ cup (50 mL) sundried tomatoes, olives and artichokes.
2. ¼ cup (50 mL) light herbed cream cheese and cooked zucchini.
3. ½ cup (125 mL) chopped asparagus with 2 tbsp. (25 mL) grated Gruyère, 2 tbsp. (25 mL) smoked salmon and tarragon to taste.
4. ¼ cup (50 mL) each chopped tomato and alfalfa sprouts or diced mushrooms.
5. 2 tbsp. (25 mL) each grated part-skim mozzarella cheese, 2% cottage cheese and sliced green onion.
6. ¼ cup (50 mL) chopped cooked vegetables and 2 tbsp. (25 mL) grated part-skim mozzarella cheese.
7. 2 tbsp. (25 mL) each 2% cottage cheese and Apple Butter (page 81).
8. 2 tsp. (10 mL) Pepperonata (page 217).

Vegetables: the mean greens machine

Portobello Mushroom Burgers with Herbed-Mustard Sauce

¼ cup	low fat mayonnaise	50 mL
¼ cup	low fat yogurt	50 mL
2 tbsp.	freshly chopped basil OR 2 tsp. (10 mL) dried	25 mL
2 tbsp.	freshly chopped parsley	25 mL
1 tbsp.	Dijon mustard	15 mL
1 tsp.	honey	5 mL
½ tsp.	salt	2 mL
½ tsp.	pepper	2 mL
1	clove garlic, minced	1
4	large Portobello mushrooms, stems removed	4
¼ cup	olive oil	50 mL
4	medium whole grain buns, split	4
4	large lettuce leaves	4
4	thick slices tomato	4

These large, meaty mushrooms make a sophisticated, meatless sandwich that's satisfying and easy to grill. Kissed with garlic, redolent of herbs, you'll enjoy these as a change from the usual.

Method

1. Whisk together mayonnaise, yogurt, basil, parsley, mustard, honey, salt, pepper and garlic.
2. Position oven rack in top third of oven. Preheat broiler.
3. Place mushrooms, stem side up, on foil-lined baking sheet. Brush with oil. Broil mushrooms until just cooked through, about 3 minutes.
4. Place bottom half of buns on serving plate. Top each with 1 mushroom, then lettuce leaf and tomato slice. Season with sauce over tomato and top with bun.

1 Serving:
Protein 7 grams
Fat 10 grams
Carbohydrate 38 grams
Calories 270

Herbed Spaghetti Squash Parmigiana

This squash is truly amazing in its likeness to strands of pasta. A nice, light accompaniment to roasted or grilled meats. This squash is also excellent served like pasta with Basic Tomato Sauce (page 214).

Makes 4 servings

1 Serving:
Protein 1 gram
Fat 2 grams
Carbohydrate 10 grams
Calories 62

1	spaghetti squash (1½–2 lb/750 g–1 kg)	1
2 tbsp.	minced parsley	25 mL
1 tbsp.	grated Parmesan cheese	15 mL
2 tsp.	butter or soft margarine	10 mL
⅛ tsp.	salt	0.5 mL
	freshly ground pepper	

Method

1. Pierce the skin of squash in several places.
2. Place on a flat microwaveable plate; **microwave** at High for 12 to 16 minutes or until pulp can easily be pierced with a fork, turning over once during cooking. Let stand for 5 minutes. Cut in half and remove seeds. OR cut squash lengthwise into quarters and remove seeds; cover with water and **cook on top of stove** until tender, about 20 minutes.
3. Using a fork, shred and separate the pulp into strands in a serving bowl.
4. Add parsley, cheese, butter, salt and pepper to taste; toss to mix well.

Spinach with Rosemary

2 tsp.	butter or soft margarine	10 mL
¼ cup	chopped onion	50 mL
½ cup	sliced mushrooms	125 mL
¼ cup	chicken stock	50 mL
¼ to ½ tsp.	fresh rosemary	1 to 2 mL
5 cups	spinach or Swiss chard leaves, washed and torn into medium pieces	1.25 L

Subtly Italian, this pleasant vegetable accompaniment has a vivid color and is a good source of iron.

Method

1. In a medium non-stick skillet, melt butter over medium heat. Add onion; sauté for 2 to 3 minutes or until softened.
2. Add mushrooms; sauté for 2 to 3 minutes or until mushrooms are tender.
3. Add chicken stock and rosemary; stir in spinach a handful at a time.
4. Cover and simmer just until spinach has wilted.
5. Remove spinach to a warm serving bowl and cover to keep warm.
6. Bring liquid remaining in skillet to a boil; cook for 2 to 3 minutes or until reduced by half.
7. Pour over spinach and serve.

Makes 2 servings

1 Serving:
Protein 3 grams
Fat 3.5 grams
Carbohydrate 4 grams
Calories 60

Rosemary is one of the oldest herbs known and is an excellent accompaniment to all manner of dishes.

Parsnip and Spinach Purée

A rich creamy green, this mixture is an excellent way to enjoy both parsnips and spinach. Hardy root vegetables, parsnips are easily available in the winter months.

1 lb	parsnips, peeled and coarsely chopped (about 4 cups/1 L)	500 g
1	10 oz (284 g) bag fresh spinach, trimmed and washed	1
4 tsp.	lemon juice	20 mL
1 tbsp.	2% milk	15 mL
1 tbsp.	butter or soft margarine	15 mL
¼ tsp.	salt	1 mL
	white pepper	

Method

1. In a medium saucepan, **boil** parsnips in water for 15 to 20 minutes or until tender; drain. OR **microwave** covered at High for 4 to 6 minutes or until tender; drain.
2. **Steam** spinach for about 5 minutes or until wilted; drain. OR **microwave** covered at High for 3 minutes until wilted; drain.
3. In food processor, purée parsnips with lemon juice, milk, butter and salt; add drained spinach and purée until well blended.
4. Season with pepper to taste.

Makes 4 servings

1 Serving:
Protein 4 grams
Fat 3 grams
Carbohydrate 25 grams
Calories 143

Minted Peas

The lettuce uniquely complements these classically flavored peas. Another bonus is the fiber content of this vegetable dish.

1 tbsp.	butter or soft margarine	15 mL
2 cups	frozen peas	500 mL
1½ cups	coarsely shredded iceberg lettuce	375 mL
½ cup	sliced green onions	125 mL
1 to 2 tbsp.	chopped fresh mint	15 to 25 mL
⅛ tsp.	freshly ground pepper	0.5 mL

Microwave Method

1. In a 2 qt. (2 L) microwaveable casserole, microwave butter at High for 30 seconds or until melted.
2. Add peas, lettuce, onions, mint and pepper; cover and microwave at High for 6 to 8 minutes or until heated through and tender, stirring once.
3. Let stand for 2 to 3 minutes.

Makes 4 servings

1 Serving:
Protein 4 grams
Fat 3 grams
Carbohydrate 10 grams
Calories 83

The ancients believed that mint aroused latent passions and prohibited its use. There are many varieties of mint, many of which grow easily and profusely in a herb garden.

Almost No-Fat Frites

2	large baking potatoes (about 1 lb/500 g)	2	
2 tsp.	olive oil	10 mL	
½ tsp.	dried oregano	2 mL	
⅛ tsp.	freshly ground pepper	0.5 mL	
	pinch salt		

So delicious, the taste will surprise you. Crisp on the outside, tender inside, these are a fun finger food.

Method

1. Scrub potatoes and cut into ½ inch (1 cm) thick slices; cut each slice into ½ inch (1 cm) wide strips and put in a bowl.
2. Add oil, oregano, pepper and salt.
3. Arrange in single layer on a baking sheet.
4. Bake in 425°F (220°C) oven for 20 to 25 minutes or until tender and browned, turning two or three times during cooking.

Optional Mediterranean Flavors: Season with any combination of cumin, coriander, cinnamon, paprika or mint to taste.

Variation

Use 2 large sweet potatoes instead of baking potatoes. Prepare as above, steps 1, 2 3. Bake in 425°F (220°C) oven for about 15 minutes or until tender and browned, turning two or three times during cooking.

Makes 2 to 3 servings

1 Serving:
Protein 3 grams
Fat 3 grams
Carbohydrate 21 grams
Calories 123

NOTE:
If preparation of potatoes is done early in day, soak in cold water and then drain well; pat dry with paper towels before tossing with oil and herbs.

Vegetable Medley

Delicately seasoned, this medley comprises healthy, appealing vegetables to team with your favorite fish.

1 tbsp.	vegetable oil	15 mL
½ cup	sliced onion	125 mL
1	clove garlic, minced	1
1 cup	chicken stock	250 mL
1 cup	green beans	250 mL
1 cup	cauliflower florets	250 mL
1 cup	peeled and thinly sliced yellow squash or carrots	250 mL
2 cups	coarsely shredded Chinese cabbage (Nappa)	500 mL
½ cup	thinly sliced sweet red pepper	125 mL
2 tsp.	soy sauce	10 mL
2 tsp.	water	10 mL
2 tsp.	cornstarch	10 mL
⅛ tsp.	crushed chili peppers (optional)	0.5 mL

Makes 4 servings

1 Serving:
Protein 2 grams
Fat 3.5 grams
Carbohydrate 10 grams
Calories 80

Method

1. In a non-stick wok or large skillet, heat oil over medium heat. Add onion and garlic; sauté for 1 to 2 minutes or until softened.
2. Add chicken stock, green beans and cauliflower; cover and simmer for 3 minutes.
3. Add squash and cook for 4 minutes.
4. Add cabbage and peppers; cook uncovered for 2 to 3 minutes or until vegetables are tender-crisp.
5. Mix soy sauce, water, cornstarch and chili peppers, if using, until smooth; stir into vegetable mixture.
6. Cook for 1 to 2 minutes or until mixture is thickened, stirring constantly.

Fennel Parmigiana

1	fennel bulb, trimmed and quartered	1
½ cup	chicken stock	125 mL
2 tsp.	olive oil	10 mL
2 tsp.	lemon juice	10 mL
2 tbsp.	grated Parmesan cheese	25 mL
	pinch ground nutmeg	
	freshly ground pepper	

With an interesting hint of licorice, fennel is an unusual but delicious vegetable to serve with pork tenderloin.

Method
1. In a medium saucepan, combine fennel and chicken stock; cover and bring to boil.
2. Reduce heat and simmer for 6 to 8 minutes or until tender.
3. Drain and arrange fennel in a shallow baking dish.
4. Drizzle oil and lemon juice over fennel; sprinkle with cheese, nutmeg and pepper to taste.
5. Broil for 3 to 4 minutes or until top is browned.

Variation
Substitute halved celery hearts for quartered fennel and adjust cooking time if necessary.

Makes 4 servings

1 Serving:
Protein 1.5 grams
Fat 3 grams
Carbohydrate 5 grams
Calories 53

Corn, Pepper and Tomato Sauté

This recipe makes excellent use of the late summer's bountiful harvest. Tomatoes and peppers offer vitamin C while corn is a great complex carbohydrate.

2 tsp.	olive oil	25 mL
1 cup	fresh or frozen corn kernels	250 mL
1	clove garlic, minced	1
1 tbsp.	chopped onion	15 mL
¼ cup	diced sweet red and/or green pepper	50 mL
½ cup	diced fresh tomato	125 mL
1 tbsp.	chopped fresh basil OR 1 tsp. (5 mL) dried	15 mL
⅛ tsp.	salt	0.5 mL
	freshly ground pepper	

Makes 2 servings

1 Serving:
Protein 3 grams
Fat 4.5 grams
Carbohydrate 22 grams
Calories 140

Method

1. In a non-stick skillet, heat oil over medium heat. Add corn, garlic and onion; sauté for 5 to 7 minutes or until corn is partially cooked.
2. Add peppers and cook for 2 to 3 minutes or until vegetables are tender-crisp, stirring constantly.
3. Stir in tomato, basil and salt.
4. Cook until heated through.
5. Season with pepper to taste.

Braised Carrots and Parsnips

2	small carrots	2	
2	small parsnips	2	
1 tbsp.	honey	15 mL	
1 tsp.	lemon juice	5 mL	
½ tsp	Dijon mustard	2 mL	
½ tsp.	curry powder	2 mL	
2 tsp.	butter or soft margarine	10 mL	
1 tbsp.	raisins	15 mL	

Method

1. Peel carrots and parsnips and cut in half lengthwise and then cut diagonally into thick slices.
2. Cover and **cook in water on top of stove** for 8 to 10 minutes or until tender-crisp; drain and reserve liquid. OR **microwave** covered with 1 tbsp. (25 mL) water at High for 5 to 6 minutes until tender-crisp; drain and reserve liquid.
3. In a small bowl, combine honey, lemon juice, mustard, curry and 1 tbsp. (15 mL) of reserved liquid.
4. In a small non-stick skillet, melt butter. Add carrots, parsnips and raisins; sauté for 2 minutes.
5. Stir in honey mixture and cook, stirring for 2 to 3 minutes or until vegetables are coated and heated through.

This recipe is as sexy as parsnips and carrots will ever get. Sweet spices and raisins are an enticing complement to the vegetables. Serve with basmati rice pilaf and poultry.

Makes 2 servings

1 Serving:
Protein 1 gram
Fat 4 grams
Carbohydrate 20 grams
Calories 120

Curry powder is a mixture of turmeric, coriander (cilantro), blackened red peppers, cumin, ginger, cinnamon and other spices.

Spiced Squash Purée

Creamy and smooth, this vegetable dish is fragrant with spices and sweetened by the apple. Squash is an excellent source of beta-carotene.

1	butternut or pepper squash (about 2 lb/1 kg)	1
1	apple, peeled, cored and chopped	1
¼ cup	chopped onion	50 mL
1 cup	water	250 mL
2 tsp.	butter or soft margarine	10 mL
1 tsp.	ground ginger	5 mL
1 tsp.	curry powder	5 mL

Makes 4 servings

1 Serving:
Protein 2 grams
Fat 2 grams
Carbohydrate 20 grams
Calories 106

Method
1. Peel and cube squash (you should have approximately 4 cups (1 L)).
2. In a medium saucepan, combine squash, apple and onion; cover with water.
3. Cover and bring to boil; cook until squash is tender, about 15 to 20 minutes.
4. Drain and transfer to food processor along with butter, ginger and curry; process until smooth. (Blender can be used to purée squash but you will have to purée in batches.)
5. Return to saucepan; heat until hot, stirring constantly.

Spring Asparagus

A pleasant spring dish, the creaminess of the sauce will easily replace any yearning for Hollandaise. This is an elegant, low fat accompaniment for poached salmon.

8 oz	fresh asparagus	250 g
⅓ cup	chicken stock	75 mL
2 tbsp.	2% plain yogurt	25 mL
1 tbsp.	light mayonnaise freshly ground pepper	15 mL

Makes 2 to 3 servings

1 Serving:
Protein 3 grams
Fat 2 grams
Carbohydrate 5 grams
Calories 50

Tip
Substitute broccoli or green beans for asparagus.

Method
1. Remove tough ends of asparagus.
2. Rinse asparagus and place in a skillet along with chicken stock; cover and **boil** for 3 to 5 minutes or just until asparagus is tender. OR **microwave** at High for 4½ to 7 minutes or until asparagus is tender.
3. Drain, reserving 2 tsp. (10 mL) of cooking liquid.
4. Mix reserved stock, yogurt and mayonnaise together.
5. Add pepper to taste; spoon over hot asparagus.

Tian

2 tbsp.	vegetable oil	25 mL
1 cup	sliced onion	250 mL
2	cloves garlic, minced	2
½ to 1 cup	chicken or beef stock	125 to 250 mL
1 cup	thickly sliced carrots	250 mL
½ cup	cubed yellow squash or turnips	125 mL
1 tsp.	dried tarragon	5 mL
1	bay leaf	1
1 cup	halved green beans	250 mL
1 cup	cauliflower pieces	250 mL
1 cup	cubed zucchini	250 mL
½ cup	sliced celery	125 mL
½ cup	sliced sweet green or red pepper	125 mL
1	large tomato, cut in eighths	1
	freshly ground pepper	

Method

1. In a large non-stick skillet, heat oil over medium heat. Add onion and garlic; sauté for 2 to 3 minutes or until softened.
2. Add ½ cup (125 mL) stock, carrots, squash, tarragon and bay leaf; cover and simmer for about 8 to 10 minutes or until vegetables are partially cooked.
3. Add beans and cauliflower; cover and simmer for 8 to 10 minutes longer adding extra stock if needed.
4. Stir in zucchini, celery and peppers; cover and cook for about 5 minutes or until vegetables are tender.
5. Stir in tomatoes and heat through.
6. Remove bay leaf. Season with pepper to taste.

A mixed vegetable stew which refers originally to the vessel in which it was cooked. Colorful and appealing, this medley is loaded with vitamins and minerals.

Makes 4 servings

1 Serving:
Protein 2.5 grams
Fat 6 grams
Carbohydrate 16 grams
Calories 128

Tumbling and similar exercises were performed around 2600 B.C. as religious rituals in China, but it was the Greeks who coined the word "gymnastics."

Caraway Cabbage

Cabbage is a choice brassica and this side dish is a pleasant complement to a menu of grilled pork chops and potato gratin.

Makes 2 servings

1 Serving:
Protein 1 gram
Fat 6 grams
Carbohydrate 5 grams
Calories 78

1 tbsp.	butter or soft margarine	15 mL
2 cups	coarsely sliced cabbage (about ¼ small head)	500 mL
1	small clove garlic, minced	1
2 tbsp.	2% plain yogurt	25 mL
¼ tsp.	granulated sugar	1 mL
¼ tsp.	caraway seeds	1 mL

Method

1. In a medium non-stick skillet, melt butter over medium heat. Add cabbage and garlic; sauté for 2 to 3 minutes or until cabbage has wilted; cover and reduce heat to low.
2. Cook for 5 to 8 minutes, stirring or shaking pan often or until cabbage is tender-crisp.
3. In a small bowl, combine yogurt, sugar and caraway seeds; stir into cabbage and serve immediately.

Romans regarded cabbage highly for its "physic" and medicinal effects. As one of the oldest cultivated vegetables, it has been popular with peasants as a low-cost source of essential nutrients.

Oven Roasted Root Vegetables

2	large baking potatoes, peeled and cut lengthwise into ½ inch (1.25 cm) thick wedges	2
4	large carrots, peeled and cut into ½ inch (1.25 cm) chunks	4
2	large turnips, peeled and cut into ½ inch (1.25 cm) wedges	2
5	cloves garlic	5
1	large red onion, peeled and cut into eighths	1
1 cup	chicken or vegetable stock	250 mL
¼ cup	wine vinegar	50 mL
¼ cup	maple syrup or honey	50 mL
2 tbsp.	vegetable oil	25 mL
¼ cup	freshly chopped rosemary OR 1 tbsp. (15 mL) dried	50 mL
4 cups	butternut squash, peeled and cut into ½ inch (1.25 cm) pieces	1 L

Method

1. Preheat oven to 425°F (220°C).
2. In bowl, combine potatoes, carrots, turnips, garlic and onion. Combine stock, vinegar, maple syrup, oil and rosemary; toss with vegetables.
3. Spread the vegetables in a large roasting pan and roast, covered, in the middle of the oven for 1 hour or until softened.
4. Add the squash to pan and toss.
5. Roast the vegetables, uncovered, shaking the pan occasionally, for 40 minutes more, or until they are tender and golden.

When company's coming, roast a capon or lean pork tenderloin and tuck these vegetables alongside. Sweetened with a hint of maple that enhances their own caramelization, these also make a delicious vegetarian entrée.

Makes about 10 cups

Serves 8 to 10

1 Serving:
Protein 4 grams
Fat 3 grams
Carbohydrate 35 grams
Calories 183

Grilled Vegetables

For an easy side dish, try cooking any combination of these vegetables over a fire that has been scattered with soaked vine clippings.

I	small eggplant	I
I	medium zucchini	I
I	medium sweet red, green, yellow or orange pepper	I
I	fennel bulb	I
I to 2 tbsp.	olive oil	15 to 25 mL
I tbsp.	chopped fresh basil or thyme OR ½ tsp (2 mL) dried	15 mL

Makes 2 to 4 servings

1 Serving:
Protein 3 grams
Fat 4 grams
Carbohydrate 12 grams
Calories 96

Method
1. Cut all vegetables in half lengthwise; core and remove seeds from peppers.
2. Mix oil with basil.
3. Brush vegetables on both sides with oil.
4. Place cut side down on barbecue grill about 4 inches (10 cm) from heat.
5. Cook for 10 minutes; turn vegetables over and cook for another 8 to 10 minutes or until tender.
6. Slice crosswise to serve.

Variations
▦ Parboil potato halves and whole carrots; brush as above and grill for about 4 to 5 minutes each side.
▦ Serve vegetables open-faced on Italian loaf with our Light Pesto Sauce (page 212) and low-fat mozzarella cheese.

Potato Gratin

2	large potatoes, peeled and sliced ¼ inch (0.5 cm) thick	2
1	small onion, sliced	1
⅔ cup	chicken or vegetable stock	150 mL
1	clove garlic, minced	1
¼ tsp.	dried thyme	1 mL
	freshly ground pepper	

Adapted from the classic French dish, we have substituted stock for cream and come up with a comforting vegetable to accompany any roast.

Method

1. In a lightly greased 1½ qt. (1.5 L) casserole, combine potatoes and onion.
2. Mix stock, garlic, thyme and pepper to taste and pour over potatoes.
3. Cover and bake in 425°F (220°C) oven for 25 to 30 minutes or until almost tender.
4. Uncover and cook until top is browned and liquid has evaporated, about 15 minutes.

Variation

Substitute sweet potatoes for white potatoes and sprinkle with ⅓ cup (75 mL) partly skimmed mozzarella cheese.

Makes 2 servings

1 Serving:
Protein 3 grams
Carbohydrate 24 grams
Calories 108

Potatoes had "unwholesome aphrodisiac effects" according to Lord Byron. However, we think potatoes are highly versatile and delicious with or without sauces. Store in a dark cool place to prevent them from turning green.

Pasta and Grains: high octane nutrition

Lentil and Brown Rice Pilaf

A combination of lentils and rice makes this the perfect, as well as eminently satisfying, non-meat dish. Rich in complex carbohydrates, our pilaf makes a great dinner the night before a 10 km run.

1 tbsp.	vegetable oil	15 mL
1	clove garlic, minced	1
½ cup	chopped onion	125 mL
¼ cup	dried green lentils, washed	50 mL
¼ cup	brown rice	50 mL
1	19 oz (540 mL) can tomatoes, mashed	1
¼ cup	beef or vegetable stock	50 mL
½ tsp.	ground coriander	2 mL
½ tsp.	ground cumin	2 mL
⅛ tsp.	salt	0.5 mL
1 tbsp.	chopped fresh coriander (cilantro) or parsley	5 mL

Method

1. In a medium non-stick saucepan, heat oil over medium heat. Add garlic and onion; sauté for 2 to 3 minutes or until softened.
2. Add lentils and rice; sauté for 3 to 4 minutes or until lightly browned.
3. Add tomatoes, beef stock, ground coriander, cumin and salt.
4. Cover and bring to boil; reduce heat and simmer for about 1 hour or until lentils are tender and liquid is absorbed.
5. Just before serving stir in fresh coriander or parsley.

Makes 2 servings

1 Serving:
Protein 9 grams
Fat 7 grams
Carbohydrate 44 grams
Calories 275

Classic Risotto (page 150)
Almost No-Fat Frites (page 149)

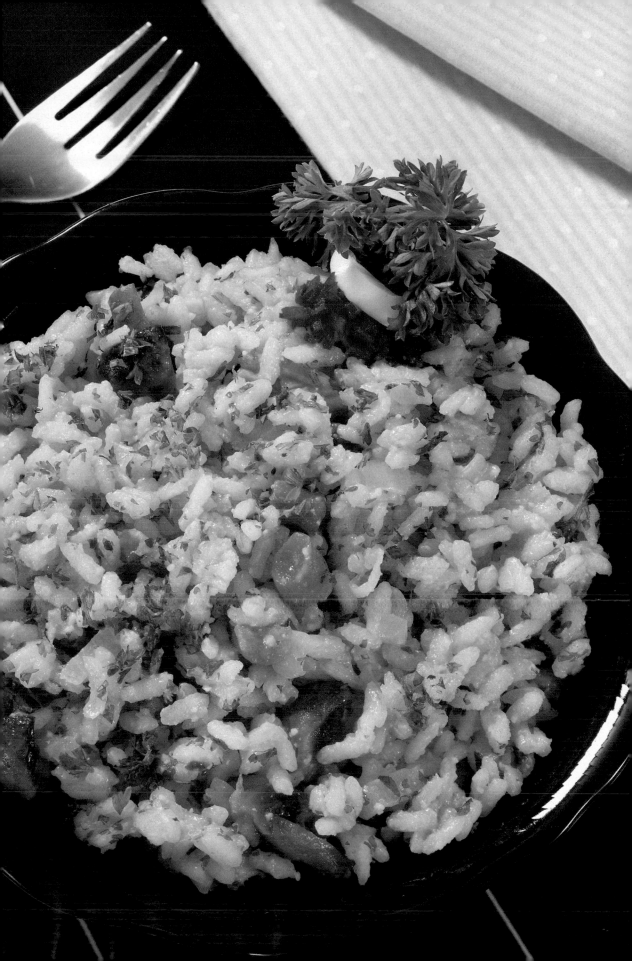

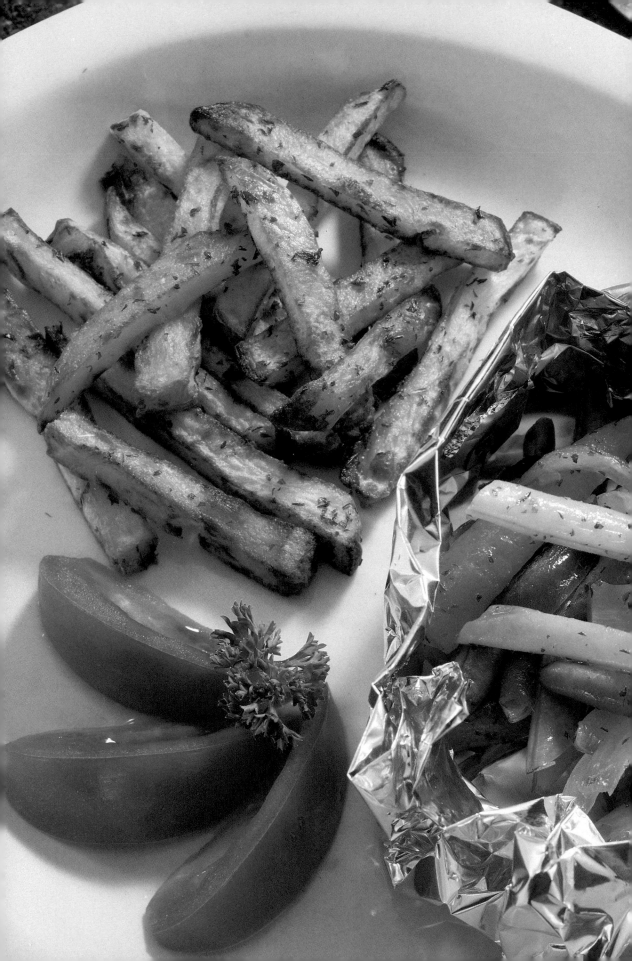

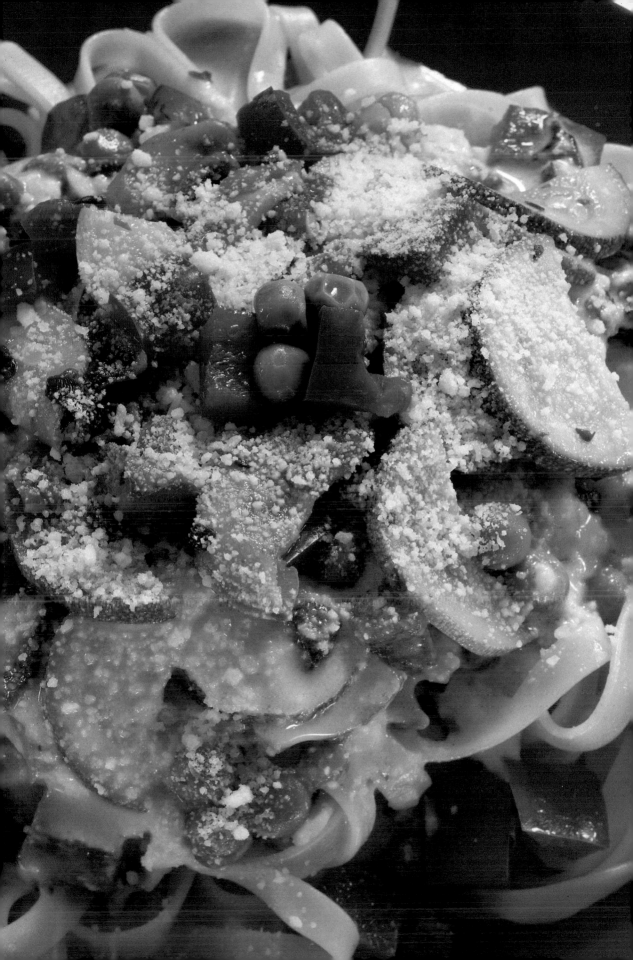

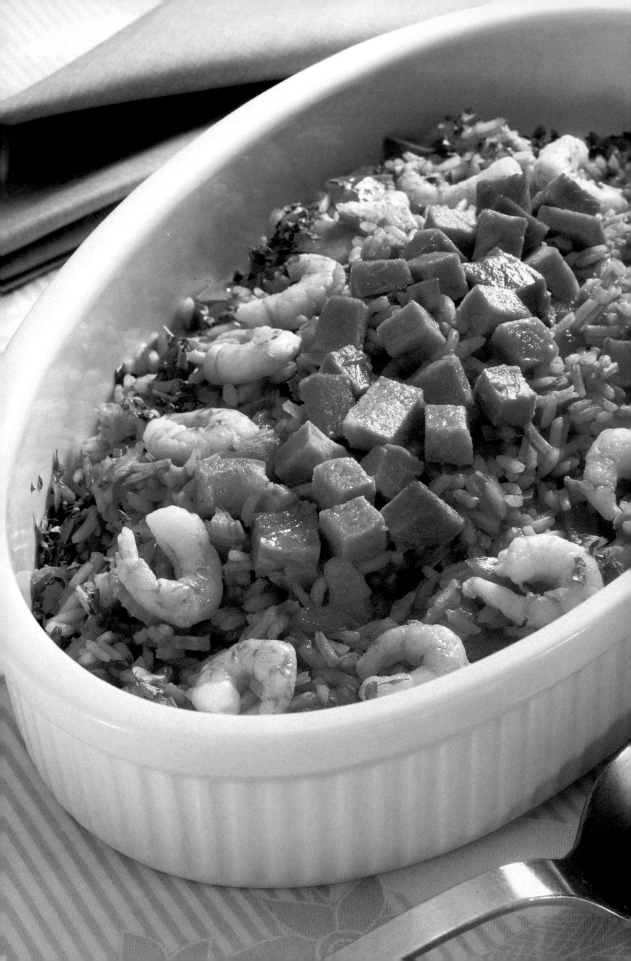

Polenta

1¾ cups	water	425 mL	
½ cup	cornmeal	125 mL	
2 tsp.	olive oil	10 mL	
¼ tsp.	salt	1 mL	
⅓ cup	grated Parmesan cheese	75 mL	
	freshly ground pepper		
	nutmeg, to taste		

Method

1. In 3 qt. (3 L) microwaveable casserole, combine water, cornmeal, oil and salt.
2. Cover and **microwave** at High for 9 to 11 minutes, stirring twice, or until thickened. OR **cook** cornmeal with 2 cups (500 mL) hot water on **top of stove**, stirring constantly until thickened.
3. Stir in cheese and season with pepper and nutmeg to taste. Serve immediately.

Variation

Grilled Polenta: Spread polenta in a loaf pan or divide between 4-10 oz (300 mL) custard cups; let stand until firm. Unmold onto baking sheet. Broil or grill for 6 to 7 minutes on each side or until browned.

Easily prepared in the microwave, this flavorful substitute for potatoes or rice is excellent alone or topped with our Bolognese (page 166) or Basic Tomato Sauce (page 214). Originally from the northern Alpine region of Italy, polenta is kind to the appetite and soul.

Makes 4 servings

1 Serving:
Protein 4 grams
Fat 5 grams
Carbohydrate 14 grams
Calories 117

Fettucine Primavera (page 163)
Creole Jambalaya (page 177)

Lemon Rice Pilaf

Pretty and perfect in
minutes, this side dish is
fragrant with citrus and a
superb partner to fish and
chicken dishes.

2 tsp.	butter or soft margarine	10 mL
¼ cup	chopped onion	50 mL
¼ cup	chopped celery	50 mL
½ cup	long-grain rice	125 mL
1 cup	chicken stock	250 mL
1 tbsp.	lemon juice	15 mL
1	½ in (1 cm) strip of lemon peel	1
1 tsp.	grated lemon rind	5 mL
1 tbsp.	fresh parsley or dill, chopped OR	15 mL
⅛ tsp.	poppy seeds	0.5 mL

Makes 2 servings

1 Serving:
Protein 4 grams
Fat 4 grams
Carbohydrate 45 grams
Calories 232

Tip
Instead of throwing away lemons
after juice is squeezed, store them
in the freezer. When grated peel is
needed, frozen peel is easy to grate.

Microwave Method

1. In a 1½ qt. (1.5 L) microwaveable casserole, combine butter, onion and celery.
2. Microwave at High for 1 minute; stir in rice and microwave at High for 3 to 4 minutes or until golden, stirring once.
3. Add chicken stock, lemon juice, strip of lemon peel; cover and microwave at High for about 4 minutes or until boiling.
4. Microwave at Medium (50%) for 6 to 8 minutes or until rice is tender and liquid is absorbed.
5. Remove lemon strip; stir in grated lemon rind and parsley or poppy seeds.
6. Let stand for 5 minutes.

Fettucine Primavera

1 tbsp.	olive oil	15 mL
1 tbsp.	minced shallots	15 mL
2 cups	sliced mushrooms	500 mL
1 cup	sliced zucchini	250 mL
½ cup	coarsely chopped sweet red or green peppers	125 mL
¼ cup	frozen peas	125 mL
1 tbsp.	water	15 mL
1 cup	Indispensable Cheese Sauce made with Parmesan cheese (page 215)	250 mL
2 tbsp.	dry white wine	25 mL
½ tsp.	ground nutmeg	2 mL
4 oz	fettucine, cooked	125 g
2 tbsp.	grated Parmesan cheese	25 mL
2 tbsp.	diced tomato (optional)	25 mL

A symphony of fresh vegetables, laced with a reduced-fat creamy sauce which rivals the traditional in satisfying good taste.

Method

1. In a large non-stick skillet, heat oil over medium heat. Add shallots; sauté for 1 to 2 minutes or until softened; add mushrooms, zucchini and peppers; sauté for 2 minutes.
2. Add peas and water; cover and steam for 2 to 3 minutes or until vegetables are tender-crisp.
3. Meanwhile, in small saucepan, heat cheese sauce until hot.
4. Stir in wine and nutmeg.
5. Toss fettucine and vegetables together.
6. Pour sauce over all and toss.
7. Sprinkle with Parmesan cheese and tomato, if using.

Makes 2 servings

1 Serving:
Protein 23 grams
Fat 21 grams
Carbohydrate 55 grams
Calories 501

Vermicelli Pescatore

This pasta dish is adapted from a "fisherman-style" richly sauced Sicilian original. Tomatoes and seafood marry for a full-bodied sauce to toss with thin spaghetti.

Makes 2 servings

1 Serving:
Protein 21 grams
Fat 1.5 grams
Carbohydrate 50 grams
Calories 297

2 cups	Basic Tomato Sauce (page 214)	500 mL
¼ cup	dry white wine or clam juice	50 mL
1 cup	frozen shrimp and/or scallops, thawed	250 mL
pinch	crushed chili peppers	pinch
	freshly ground pepper	
4 oz	vermicelli, cooked	125 g
	minced parsley for garnish	

Method

1. In a medium saucepan, heat tomato sauce and wine over medium heat until hot.
2. Stir in seafood; cover and cook until shrimp turn pink or scallops are opaque, about 3 minutes. Season with chilies and pepper to taste.
3. Spoon vermicelli onto plates and top with seafood sauce.
4. Sprinkle parsley over top.

Spaghetti with Tuna and Tomato Sauce

1 tbsp.	olive oil	15 mL
¼ cup	chopped onion	50 mL
1	clove garlic, minced	1
1 cup	sliced mushrooms (about 2 oz/60 g)	250 mL
1	19 oz (540 mL) can tomatoes, broken	1
2 tbsp.	capers	25 mL
1	6.5 oz (184 g) can tuna, packed in water, drained and flaked	1
	freshly ground pepper	
6 oz	spaghetti, cooked	180 g

Method
1. In a medium non-stick saucepan, heat oil over medium heat. Add onion and garlic; sauté for 3 to 4 minutes or until softened.
2. Stir in mushrooms; sauté for 2 minutes.
3. Add tomatoes and capers; bring to boil.
4. Reduce heat to medium and cook for 3 to 5 minutes or until thickened slightly.
5. Stir in tuna and season with pepper to taste.
6. Toss with spaghetti.

Variation
Substitute 1 can (10 oz/283 g) baby clams for tuna and garnish with 2 tbsp. (25 mL) grated Parmesan cheese.

After a day at the office and a session on the weights, no dish could be simpler, quicker or more tasty. Stirred together in minutes, these ingredients can be kept on hand for a nourishing meal-in-a-flash.

Makes 3 servings

1 Serving:
Protein 28 grams
Fat 5 grams
Carbohydrate 39 grams
Calories 313

Capers are often confused with nasturtium buds. These tiny flower buds packed in salt or vinegar originate from their very own edible bush in the Mediterranean.

Spaghetti Bolognese

Our rich and aromatic version of this classic meat sauce from Bologna serves up equally well over pasta or polenta.

1 tbsp.	olive oil	15 mL
1	clove garlic, minced	1
½ cup	chopped onion	125 mL
½ cup	chopped celery	125 mL
¼ cup	finely chopped carrot	50 mL
5 oz	lean ground beef	166 g
¼ tsp.	freshly ground pepper	1 mL
⅛ tsp.	salt	0.5 mL
pinch	ground nutmeg	pinch
½ cup	dry red or white wine	125 mL
¾ cup	beef stock	175 mL
1 tbsp.	tomato paste	15 mL
¼ cup	canned 2% evaporated milk	50 mL
	freshly ground pepper	
4 oz	spaghetti, cooked	125 g

Makes 2 servings

1 Serving:
Protein 23 grams
Fat 17 grams
Carbohydrate 39 grams
Calories 401

Tip
Low fat canned evaporated milk is a convenient way to add rich creaminess to a dish without adding much butterfat.

Method

1. In a medium non-stick skillet or saucepan, heat oil over medium heat. Add garlic, onion, celery and carrot; sauté for 3 to 4 minutes or until softened.
2. Add ground beef, pepper, salt and nutmeg; cook for about 5 minutes or until browned, stirring constantly to crumble beef.
3. Add wine and cook for about 5 minutes or until moisture evaporates.
4. Stir in beef stock and tomato paste; bring to boil.
5. Reduce heat; cover and simmer for about 30 minutes or until slightly thickened, stirring occasionally.
6. Stir in milk. Adjust seasoning with pepper to taste.
7. Spoon spaghetti onto plates and top with meat sauce.

Orecchetti with Broccoli Anchovy Sauce

1	broccoli stalk, including florets	1	
2 tsp.	olive oil	10 mL	
¼ cup	chopped onion	50 mL	
1	small clove garlic, minced	1	
2	flat anchovies, drained, rinsed and chopped	2	
⅓ cup	chicken stock	75 mL	
2 oz	orecchetti, cooked	60 g	
2 tbsp.	freshly grated Parmesan cheese, divided	2	
5 mL	freshly ground pepper		

These "little ears" of pasta catch the rich flavors from a vibrant and robust sauce. No recipe could be simpler than this combination of pasta and a brassica vegetable.

Method

1. Separate broccoli into florets; peel stem and slice thinly.
2. **Blanch** the broccoli in boiling water until tender-crisp, about 3 minutes. OR **microwave** at High for about 2 minutes; drain.
3. Plunge into cold water to chill; drain.
4. In a small non-stick skillet or saucepan, heat oil over medium heat. Add onion and garlic; sauté for 2 to 3 minutes or until softened; add anchovies and mash into onion mixture.
5. Add chicken stock; bring to boil and cook for 2 minutes.
6. Add broccoli; heat until hot.
7. Toss with orecchetti and half the cheese.
8. Season with pepper to taste and sprinkle remaining cheese over top.

Makes 1 serving

1 Serving:
Protein 14 grams
Fat 14 grams
Carbohydrate 40 grams
Calories 342

Fusilli with Artichokes and Red Peppers

Topped with pine nuts, this sauce is a simple pleasant sauté of artichoke hearts and peppers.

1 tbsp.	olive oil	15 mL
½ cup	sliced onion	125 mL
1	small clove garlic, minced	1
½	sweet red pepper, thinly sliced	½
½ cup	chicken stock	125 mL
2 tsp.	red wine vinegar	10 mL
½ cup	sliced canned artichoke bottoms (about 2 large)	125 mL
2 tbsp.	chopped fresh parsley	25 mL
2 tsp.	fresh rosemary OR ½ tsp (2 mL) dried	10 mL
4 oz	fusilli, cooked	125 g
2 tbsp.	toasted pine nuts	25 mL

Makes 2 servings

1 Serving (with pine nuts):
Protein 8 grams
Fat 11 grams
Carbohydrate 40 grams
Calories 291

Tip

To Toast Pine Nuts: Spread pine nuts on a pie plate and bake in 350°F (180°C) oven for 5 to 10 minutes or until golden, stirring once.

Method

1. In a medium non-stick skillet, heat olive oil over medium heat. Add onion and garlic; sauté for 3 to 4 minutes or until softened. Add red pepper; sauté for 2 minutes.
2. Add chicken stock and vinegar; simmer for 2 to 3 minutes or until peppers are tender.
3. Stir in artichokes, parsley and rosemary; simmer until heated through.
4. Toss with fusilli and sprinkle pine nuts over top.

Spaghettini with Oriental Vegetables

1 to 2	dried Chinese mushrooms	1 to 2
2 tsp.	vegetable oil	10 mL
1	onion, peeled and cut in wedges	1
1	clove garlic, minced	1
1 tsp.	minced fresh gingerroot	5 mL
1 cup	julienned carrot	250 mL
1 cup	julienned Japanese white radish	250 mL
1 cup	julienned zucchini	250 mL
⅔ cup	chicken stock	150 mL
1 cup	bean sprouts	250 mL
pinch	crushed chili peppers	pinch
1 tbsp.	lemon juice	15 mL
1 tbsp.	soy sauce	15 mL
1 tsp.	water	5 mL
1 tsp.	cornstarch	5 mL
4 oz	spaghettini, cooked	125 g

Method

1. Soak Chinese mushrooms in very hot water for 30 minutes.
2. Rinse and cut away the woody stems. Rinse again and slice thinly.
3. In a large non-stick skillet, heat oil over medium heat. Add onion, garlic and gingerroot; sauté for 2 to 3 minutes or until onion has softened.
4. Add carrot, radish, zucchini and chicken stock; cover and simmer for 3 to 5 minutes or until vegetables are tender-crisp.
5. Add bean sprouts, soaked mushrooms and chili peppers.
6. In a separate bowl, blend lemon juice, soy sauce, water and cornstarch until smooth; stir into stock and vegetables.
7. Cook, stirring constantly for about 1 minute or until thickened.
8. Toss with spaghettini.

Interesting and different crisp vegetables plus delicate Oriental seasonings make this a fabulous update of the stir-fry.

Makes 2 servings

1 Serving:
Protein 7 grams
Fat 5 grams
Carbohydrate 46 grams
Calories 257

Drying intensifies the smoky, musky flavor of Chinese mushrooms such as Cloud Ears or Tree Ears. Looking much like dried black chips before soaking, they often expand to six times their size to resemble double petunias.

Egg Bows with Sauce Forestière

Rich and exotic tasting, the full-bodied taste of the wild mushroom makes this an eminently satisfying first course.

1 oz	dried porcini mushrooms	30 g
1 tbsp.	olive oil	15 mL
1 tbsp.	minced shallots	15 mL
1½ cups	fresh mushrooms (about 4 oz/125 g)	375 mL
2 tbsp.	sherry or marsala	25 mL
2 tbsp.	canned 2% evaporated milk	25 mL
¼ tsp.	salt	2 mL
	freshly ground pepper	
4 oz	egg bows (farfel), cooked	125 g
2 tbsp.	minced fresh parsley	25 mL

Makes 4 appetizer portions

1 Portion:
Protein 4 grams
Fat 4 grams
Carbohydrates 18 grams
Calories 124

Method

1. Soak dried mushrooms in ½ cup (125 mL) warm water for 30 minutes.
2. Strain liquid through paper toweling inside a sieve and reserve; rinse mushrooms under cold running water to remove grit and thinly slice.
3. In a non-stick skillet, heat oil over medium heat; add shallots and sauté for 1 to 2 minutes or until softened.
4. Add fresh mushrooms; sauté for 2 to 3 minutes or until tender.
5. Add porcini mushrooms, reserved mushroom liquid, sherry and milk.
6. Bring to boil and cook for 3 to 4 minutes or until slightly thickened.
7. Season with salt and pepper.
8. Toss with egg bows.
9. Sprinkle parsley over top.

Porcini have a meaty flavor that becomes more intense with drying. Italian for "little pigs," these mushrooms reconstitute quickly to add their earthy flavor to soups, sauces and dressings.

Falafel

1	19 oz (540 mL) can chickpeas, drained	1
4	cloves garlic, sliced	4
1	egg	1
¼ cup	minced parsley	50 mL
3	green onions, chopped	3
¼ cup	tahini (sesame paste)	50 mL
¼ cup	dry bread crumbs	50 mL
1 tbsp.	ground cumin	15 mL
1½ tsp.	dried basil	7 mL
1½ tsp.	dried marjoram	7 mL
1½ tsp.	dried thyme	7 mL
1½ tsp.	tumeric	7 mL
¼ tsp.	freshly ground pepper	1 mL
⅛ tsp.	salt	0.5 mL
1 tbsp.	vegetable oil	15 mL
4	whole wheat pitas	4
	Tahini Sauce (see below) for topping	
	shredded iceberg lettuce for topping	
	chopped tomatoes, diced cucumbers or alfalfa sprouts for toppings	

The chickpeas provide protein and fiber in this meatless Middle Eastern burger.

Method

1. In food processor, combine the chickpeas and garlic; process until smooth.
2. Add egg and process to mix well.
3. Transfer to a medium bowl and stir in parsley, onions, tahini, bread crumbs, cumin, basil, marjoram, thyme, tumeric, pepper and salt.
4. Shape mixture into 8 (¼ inch/0.5 cm thick) patties.
5. In a large non-stick skillet, heat oil over medium-high heat; add patties and cook for 5 to 7 minutes per side or until golden brown.
6. Cut each pita in half horizontally.
7. Tuck a patty into a pita half. Pass bowls of toppings separately.

Tahini Sauce: In a small bowl combine 1 cup (250 mL) 2% plain yogurt, 2 tbsp. (25 mL) tahini (sesame paste), 2 tbsp. (25 mL) minced parsley, 1 tbsp. (15 mL) lemon juice, 2 green onions (minced), 1 clove garlic (minced), ½ tsp. (2 mL) ground cumin, ⅛ tsp. (0.5 mL) freshly ground pepper, a pinch of cayenne and a pinch of salt; mix well. Cover and refrigerate for 30 minutes or overnight.

Makes 4 servings

1 Serving (with Tahini Sauce):
Protein 23 grams
Fat 17 grams
Carbohydrate 69 grams
Calories 521

Louisiana Rice and Beans

For a hearty Cajun menu high in complex carbohydrates, serve this side dish with Blackened Pork Chops (page 188). If you're celebrating after a great afternoon on the slopes, chase this down with a cold beer.

½ cup	finely chopped onion	125 mL
1	small clove garlic, minced	1
¾ cup	beef stock	175 mL
1	14 oz (398 mL) can red kidney beans, drained and rinsed	1
1 cup	cooked rice	250 mL
½ cup	chopped sweet green peppers	125 mL
1 tsp.	Worcestershire sauce	5 mL
½ tsp.	dried oregano	2 mL
¼ tsp.	pepper	1 mL
¼ tsp.	chili powder	1 mL
⅛ tsp.	salt	0.5 mL
dash	hot pepper sauce	dash
2 tbsp.	chopped red onion (optional)	25 mL

Method

1. In a medium saucepan, combine onion, garlic and beef stock; cover and bring to boil.
2. Reduce heat and simmer for 8 to 10 minutes or until onion has softened.
3. Stir in kidney beans, rice, green pepper, Worcestershire sauce, oregano, pepper, chili powder, salt and hot pepper sauce.
4. Simmer until hot.
5. Top with chopped red onion, if using.

Makes 2 servings

1 Serving:
Protein 14 grams
Fat 1 gram
Carbohydrate 60 grams
Calories 305

▦   ▦   ▦   ▦   ▦   ▦   ▦

The Big Easy Menu

Tri-Color Pepper Salad (page 113)

Blackened Pork Chops (page 188)

Louisiana Rice and Beans

Fresh Fruit Brulé (page 232)

These large beans, so called for their kidney-like shape and reddish color, are most familiar in chili. Keep a few cans on hand for a quick protein boost to meatless main dishes or salads.

Spicy Thai Noodles

½ package	125 g package wide Chinese rice noodles or rice vermicelli	25 mL
¼ cup	Asian fish sauce or soy sauce	50 mL
2 tbsp.	tomato paste	25 mL
2 tbsp.	rice vinegar	25 mL
2 tbsp.	brown sugar	25 mL
¼ tsp.	cayenne	1 mL
2	large eggs, lightly beaten	2
1 tbsp.	vegetable oil	15 mL
3	cloves garlic, minced	3
½ lb	shrimp, peeled and deveined	250 g
16 oz	firm tofu, chopped	500 g
½ cup	mint leaves	125 mL
½ cup	coriander leaves	125 mL
½ cup	basil leaves	125 mL
4	green onions, thinly sliced on the diagonal	4
¼ cup	lime juice	50 mL
½ cup	chopped roasted peanuts (optional)	125 mL
	coriander (cilantro) sprigs for garnish	
	lime wedges for garnish	

If you've never made a Thai dish before, this is a great one to start with. Easy to make, richly flavorful and perfect for vegetarians.

Method

1. In a large bowl soak noodles in hot water until they are softened, about 15 minutes. Drain.
2. In a small bowl stir together fish sauce, tomato paste, vinegar, brown sugar and cayenne.
3. In a non-stick skillet over medium heat, add eggs, and cook, stirring until they are set and just cooked through. Transfer to a bowl and break into pieces.
4. In the same pan, heat oil over medium heat. Add garlic, shrimp and tofu; stir-fry for 3 minutes or until shrimp are pink and opaque.
5. Add tomato paste mixture, noodles and ½ cup water. Bring to a boil; cook until the liquid has reduced slightly, about 1 minute.
6. Add egg, mint, coriander, basil, green onion and lime juice and toss together.
7. To serve, place on a serving platter and garnish with peanuts, coriander sprigs and lime wedges.

4 servings

1 Serving:
Protein 41 grams
Fat 15 grams
Carbohydrate 40 grams
Calories 459

Garden Lasagna

Always a favorite with a hungry crowd, this hearty meatless main course can be prepared ahead and simply reheated in the microwave.

1 tbsp.	olive oil	15 mL
½ cup	chopped onion	125 mL
1	clove garlic, minced	1
1½ cups	sliced mushrooms	375 mL
1	28 oz (796 mL) can tomatoes, crushed	1
1	19 oz (540 mL) can tomatoes, crushed	1
1 tbsp.	dried basil OR ¼ cup (50 mL) fresh	15 mL
1 tbsp.	dried parsley OR ¼ cup (50 mL) fresh	15 mL
¼ tsp.	salt	1 mL
¼ tsp.	pepper	1 mL
1	10 oz (300 g) package, frozen chopped spinach, thawed and drained	1
1½ cups	ricotta cheese	375 mL
½ cup	grated Parmesan cheese, divided	125 mL
1	egg	1
¼ cup	chopped sweet red pepper or pimento	50 mL
2 tbsp.	2% milk	25 mL
¼ tsp.	nutmeg	1 mL
6	oven-ready or no-boil lasagna noodles	6
2 cups	sliced zucchini (about 1 medium)	500 mL
1½ cups	grated part-skim mozzarella cheese, divided	375 mL

Method

1. In a large non-stick saucepan, heat oil over medium heat. Add onion and garlic; sauté for 2 to 3 minutes or until softened.
2. Add mushrooms; sauté for 2 minutes.
3. Add both cans of tomatoes; stir in basil, parsley, salt and pepper.
4. Bring to boil; reduce heat and simmer uncovered for 20 minutes.
5. Meanwhile, squeeze moisture from spinach; combine with ricotta cheese, ⅓ cup (75 mL) of the Parmesan cheese, egg, red pepper, milk and nutmeg.
6. Spread a thin layer of tomato sauce in a lightly greased 9 x 13 inch (3.5 L) baking dish.
7. Arrange 3 lasagna noodles in single layer over tomato sauce.
8. Spread one-half of ricotta mixture over noodles.
9. Cover with one-half zucchini; sprinkle with ½ cup (125 mL) of the mozzarella cheese.
10. Spoon a layer of tomato sauce over cheese.
11. Repeat layers ending with remaining tomato sauce.

Makes 8 servings

1 Serving:
Protein 19 grams
Fat 12 grams
Carbohydrate 34 grams
Calories 320

12. Cover and bake in 325°F (160°C) oven for 45 to 60 minutes or until noodles are almost tender.

13. Uncover and sprinkle with remaining Parmesan and mozzarella cheese.

14. Return to oven and bake for 10 to 15 minutes or until cheese has melted.

15. Let stand for 10 minutes before cutting to serve.

Fettucine with a Trio of Cheeses

⅓ cup	2% cottage cheese	75 mL
⅓ cup	light cream cheese	75 mL
⅓ cup	crumbled blue cheese	75 mL
2 tbsp.	2% milk	25 mL
½ cup	finely chopped tomatoes	125 mL
4 oz	fettucine, cooked	125 g
	freshly ground pepper	

Tangy and pungent from blue cheese, this creamy sauce is reduced in fat yet still scores a hit with hungry athletes.

Method

1. In blender or food processor, combine cottage cheese, cream cheese, blue cheese and milk; process until smooth.

2. Pour into heavy saucepan and heat over low heat until cheeses have melted.

3. Just before serving, stir in tomatoes.

4. Toss with pasta and season with pepper to taste.

Makes 2 servings

1 Serving:
Protein 19 grams
Fat 14 grams
Carbohydrate 37 grams
Calories 350

Penne with Arrabbiata Sauce

Piquant rather than the "angry" that arrabbiata literally means, red chilies and garlic combine for an intensely flavored sauce.

1 tsp.	olive oil	125 mL
2 tbsp.	chopped onion	25 mL
1	small clove garlic, minced	1
1	medium tomato, peeled and chopped	1
1 tbsp.	chopped fresh parsley	25 mL
⅛ tsp.	salt	0.5 mL
pinch to ⅛ tsp.	crushed chili peppers	0.5 mL
	freshly ground pepper	
2 oz	penne, cooked	60 g
2 tbsp.	freshly grated Parmesan cheese (optional)	25 mL

Method

1. In a small non-stick skillet, heat oil over medium heat. Add onion and garlic; sauté for 2 to 3 minutes or until softened.
2. Add tomatoes, parsley, salt, chili peppers and pepper to taste.
3. Cook for 2 to 3 minutes.
4. Toss with cooked penne.
5. Sprinkle with cheese, if using.

Makes 1 serving

1 Serving (without cheese):
Protein 6 grams
Fat 5 grams
Carbohydrate 37 grams
Calories 217

Creole Jambalaya

1 tbsp.	vegetable oil	15 mL
½ cup	chopped green pepper	125 mL
½ cup	chopped celery	125 mL
¼ cup	chopped green onion	50 mL
1	clove garlic, minced	1
1	14 oz (398 mL) can tomatoes, broken up	1
½ cup	water	125 mL
1	bay leaf	1
⅛ tsp.	dried thyme	0.5 mL
⅛ tsp.	cayenne	0.5 mL
⅛ tsp.	freshly ground pepper	0.5 mL
⅛ tsp.	salt	0.5 mL
½ cup	long-grain rice	125 mL
½ cup	diced cooked ham	125 mL
4 oz	frozen shrimp, thawed	125 g
2 tbsp.	chopped fresh parsley	25 mL

Method

1. In a medium non-stick saucepan, heat oil over medium heat. Add green pepper, celery, green onion and garlic; sauté for 2 to 3 minutes or until softened.
2. Add tomatoes, water, bay leaf, thyme, cayenne, pepper and salt; bring to boil.
3. Stir in rice; cover and reduce heat. Simmer, stirring occasionally until rice is tender, about 20 minutes.
4. Add ham and shrimp; cook for 2 to 3 minutes longer or until shrimp turns pink.
5. Stir in parsley.

Robustly seasoned and smoky-flavored, this one-dish entrée owes its origins to the Deep South. High in complex carbohydrates and protein, this dish is guaranteed to take the chill off any skier's bones in a hurry.

Makes 2 servings

1 Serving:
Protein 27 grams
Fat 9 grams
Carbohydrate 54 grams
Calories 405

Long-grain white rice is the most common rice in Canada and the United States. The outer hull and bran have been removed in the processing. Some long-grain rice is parboiled or called "converted" by manufacturers. It produces a firmer and more separate grain than instant or pre-cooked rice and is more nutritious.

Short-grain white rice produces a stickier rice which is good to eat with chopsticks. Use it to make rice pudding or risotto.

Vegetarian Chili

Wonderfully hot, this "just right" spiced meatless version is great alone or as a topping on baked potatoes or Sesame Corn Bread (page 230). Protein and complex carbohydrates make this a good low fat choice for any athletes concerned about their diet.

1 tbsp.	olive oil	15 mL
1 cup	chopped celery	250 mL
1 cup	finely chopped carrot	250 mL
½ cup	chopped onion	125 mL
1	clove garlic, minced	1
1	28 oz (796 mL) can tomatoes	1
2 tbsp.	chili powder	25 mL
1 tsp.	dried oregano	5 mL
½ tsp.	ground cumin	2 mL
1½ cups	coarsely chopped zucchini or cabbage	375 mL
1 cup	chopped sweet red or green pepper	250 mL
1 cup	sliced mushrooms	250 mL
1	19 oz (540 mL) can kidney beans, undrained	1
1	19 oz (540 mL) can chickpeas, drained	1

Makes 6 servings

1 Serving:
Protein 13 grams
Fat 4 grams
Carbohydrate 45 grams
Calories 268

Method

1. In a large saucepan, heat oil over medium heat. Add celery, carrot, onion and garlic; sauté for 3 to 4 minutes or until softened; add tomatoes, chili powder, oregano and cumin.
2. Bring to boil; reduce heat and simmer for about 20 minutes, stirring occasionally.
3. Add zucchini, peppers, mushrooms, kidney beans and chickpeas; simmer for 15 to 20 minutes or until thickened.

Serving Suggestion

Taco Salad: Spoon chili over shredded iceberg lettuce and garnish with diced green onions, tomatoes, green peppers, 2% plain yogurt and grated Cheddar cheese.

Moroccan Couscous

2 tsp.	vegetable oil	10 mL
½ cup	chopped onion	125 mL
2	cloves garlic, minced	2
1 tsp.	minced fresh gingerroot	5 mL
1½ cups	chicken stock	375 mL
1 cup	cubed butternut squash	250 mL
1 cup	sliced carrots	250 mL
½ tsp.	freshly ground pepper	2 mL
½ tsp.	ground coriander (cilantro)	2 mL
¼ to ½ tsp.	crushed chili peppers	1 to 2 mL
¼ tsp.	salt	1 mL
1	medium zucchini, cut into bite-sized pieces	1
1	19 oz (540 mL) can chickpeas, undrained	1
1	medium tomato, cut in large chunks	1
¼ cup	raisins (optional)	50 mL
¼ cup	chopped fresh parsley	50 mL
¾ cup	medium grain couscous	175 mL

This meatless main dish is a super source of protein, vitamins, minerals and fiber. Excitement in the taste is generated by the traditional Moroccan seasonings, especially the chilies.

Method

1. In a large non-stick saucepan, heat oil over medium heat. Add onion, garlic and ginger; sauté for 1 to 2 minutes or until softened.
2. Add chicken stock, squash, carrots, pepper, coriander, chili peppers and salt; cover and bring to boil.
3. Reduce heat and simmer until vegetables are tender-crisp, about 5 to 7 minutes.
3. Add zucchini and chickpeas; cook until zucchini is tender-crisp, about 2 to 3 minutes.
4. Stir in tomato, raisins, if using, and parsley.
5. Taste and adjust seasonings with chilies and pepper.
6. Meanwhile, in a separate bowl, pour ¾ cup (175 mL) boiling water over couscous; cover and let stand for 5 minutes.
7. Fluff with a fork and spoon onto individual plates or bowls.
8. Spoon vegetable mixture over couscous.

Makes 3 to 4 servings

1 Serving:
Protein 12 grams
Fat 5 grams
Carbohydrate 53 grams
Calories 305

Made from finely ground durum wheat that is steamed and dried, couscous is a convenience grain that is quickly plumped in boiling water or stock.

Classic Risotto

Instead of standing stirring this creamy dish at your stove, use the microwave to make this a cinch to prepare. Serve as an appetizer or entrée; your athletic friends will love it.

½ cup	chopped onion	125 mL
1 tsp.	olive oil	5 mL
1	small clove garlic, minced	1
1¾ cups	chicken stock	425 mL
¾ cup	Italian short-grain rice (e.g., Arborio)	175 mL
pinch	saffron (optional)	pinch
2 tbsp.	dry white wine (optional)	25 mL
1½ cups	quartered mushrooms	375 mL
¼ cup	grated Parmesan cheese	50 mL
¼ cup	chopped fresh parsley	50 mL

Makes 4 servings

1 Serving:
Protein 5 grams
Fat 3 grams
Carbohydrate 32 grams
Calories 175

Microwave Method

1. In a 3 qt. (3 L) microwaveable casserole, combine onion, oil and garlic. Microwave at High for 1 minute stirring once or until onion has softened.
2. Stir in chicken stock, rice, saffron and wine, if using.
3. Microwave covered at High for 4 to 8 minutes or until boiling.
4. Stir in mushrooms and microwave covered at Medium (50%) for 6 to 9 minutes or just until rice is tender and mixture is still creamy.
5. Stir in cheese; let stand for 5 to 10 minutes.
6. Stir in parsley. Serve immediately.

Variations

Risotto with Peas: Omit mushrooms and parsley and stir in 1 cup (250 mL) thawed frozen peas with cheese.
Risotto with Asparagus: Omit mushrooms and parsley and stir in 1 cup (250 mL) cooked asparagus pieces, with the cheese.
Risotto with Seafood: Omit mushrooms. Cook as in recipe. After mixture has cooked at Medium (50%) for 5 minutes stir in 8 oz (250 g) frozen and thawed shrimps or scallops. Continue as in recipe.

Apricot Bulgar Pilaf

2 tsp.	butter or soft margarine	10 mL
2 tbsp.	minced celery	25 mL
1 tbsp.	minced onion	15 mL
1	clove garlic, minced	1
½ cup	bulgar	125 mL
1¼ cups	chicken stock	300 mL
¼ cup	sliced dried apricots	50 mL
½ tsp.	curry powder	2 mL
1 tbsp.	chopped fresh parsley or mint	15 mL

Method

1. In a medium non-stick saucepan, melt butter over medium heat. Add celery, onion and garlic; sauté for about 3 minutes or until softened.
2. Add bulgar and sauté for about 5 minutes, stirring constantly until golden brown.
3. Add chicken stock, apricots and curry powder; cover and bring to boil.
4. Reduce heat and simmer for about 10 minutes or until liquid is absorbed and bulgar is tender.
5. Stir in parsley or mint.

Bulgar is a quick-cooking, nutty-tasting whole grain, and the dried fruit in this recipe makes it a particularly flavorful side dish. Dried apricots provide beta-carotene, iron and fiber.

Makes 2 to 3 servings

1 Serving:
Protein 4 grams
Fat 3 grams
Carbohydrate 29 grams
Calories 159

The "rice" of the Middle East is cracked wheat or bulgar. Cracked into small pieces after it has been parboiled (steamed and dried), bulgar has a unique nutty flavor.

Barley Pilaf

The perfect complement for broiled meats or chicken, this pilaf is an appealing change from rice.

2 tsp.	vegetable oil	10 mL
¾ cup	finely chopped carrot	175 mL
¼ cup	chopped onion	50 mL
1½ cups	chicken stock	375 mL
½ cup	barley	125 mL
2 tbsp.	chopped fresh parsley	25 mL
½ tsp.	dried basil	2 mL
¼ tsp.	freshly ground pepper	1 mL

Makes 2 to 3 servings

1 Serving:
Protein 3 grams
Fat 3 grams
Carbohydrate 32 grams
Calories 167

Method

1. In a medium non-stick saucepan, heat oil over medium heat. Add carrot and onion; sauté for 2 to 3 minutes or until softened.
2. Stir in chicken stock and barley; cover and bring to boil.
3. Reduce heat and simmer for 45 to 55 minutes or until barley is tender and most of the liquid is absorbed.
4. Stir in parsley, basil and pepper.

Linguine with Eggplant-Tomato Sauce

2 tbsp.	olive oil	25 mL
¼ cup	chopped onion	50 mL
1	clove garlic, minced	1
½	egglant, peeled and cubed (about 2¼ cups/550 mL)	½
2	large tomatoes, peeled and coarsely chopped OR 1 14 oz (398 mL) can	2
1	sweet red pepper, sliced	1
½ cup	sliced mushrooms	125 mL
1 tsp.	chopped fresh basil OR ¼ tsp. (1 mL) dried	5 mL
1 tsp.	chopped fresh oregano OR ¼ tsp. (1 mL) dried	5 mL
¼ tsp.	salt	1 mL
	freshly ground pepper	
⅓ cup	grated Parmesan or Romano cheese, divided	75 mL
4 oz	linguine, cooked	125 g

A flavorful, economical meatless meal, this pasta dish is similar to ratatouille with the added benefit of complex carbohydrates.

Method

1. In medium non-stick saucepan, heat oil over moderate heat. Add onion, garlic and eggplant; sauté, stirring often for 5 to 8 minutes or until eggplant is tender.
2. Add tomatoes, pepper, mushrooms, basil and oregano; stir well and simmer uncovered for 15 to 20 minutes or until thickened slightly.
3. Season with salt and pepper to taste.
4. Stir in half the cheese.
5. Spoon sauce over hot pasta.
6. Sprinkle with remaining cheese.

Makes 2 main course servings or 4 appetizer servings

1 Serving (Main Dish):
Protein 13 grams
Fat 17 grams
Carbohydrate 54 grams
Calories 421

How To Cook Rice

General Directions: Add rice to boiling water; cover and cook on low according to time given or until liquid is absorbed. Let stand for 5 minutes.

Type of rice	Amount	Water	Cooking Time	Yield
Long-Grain White Rice	1 cup (250 mL) Makes 4 to 5 servings	2 cups (500 mL)	15 to 20 min.	3 cups (750 mL)
Short-Grain White Rice	1 cup (250 mL) Makes 4 to 5 servings	1¼ cups (300 mL)	15 to 20 min.	3 cups (750 mL)
Brown Rice	1 cup (250 mL) Makes 4 to 5 servings	3 cups (750 mL)	45 min. (drain off excess liquid)	3 cups (750 mL)
Wild Rice	½ cup (125 mL) Makes 3 to 4 servings	2 cups (500 mL)	40 to 45 min.	2 cups (500 mL)
Basmati Rice	1 cup (250 mL) Makes 4 to 5 servings	2 cups (500 mL)	15 to 20 min.	3 cups (750 mL)

Microwave Method for Long- or Short-Grain White: (Time isn't shortened since rice needs time to rehydrate, but it is a very easy and convenient method).

In a 3 qt. (3 L) microwaveable casserole, combine 1 cup (250 mL) rice and 2 cups (500 mL) water. Cover and microwave at High until boiling, about 4 to 7 minutes; then microwave at Medium (50%) for 10 to 12 minutes or until rice is tender and most of the water has been absorbed. Let stand for 10 minutes.

Microwave Method for Brown Rice: In a 3 qt. (3 L) casserole combine 1 cup (250 mL) rice and 2½ cups (625 mL) water. Cover and microwave at High for 4 to 7 minutes or until boiling; then microwave at Medium (50%) for 25 to 35 minutes or until rice is tender and most of the water has been absorbed. Let stand for 10 minutes.

Tip

Extra cooked rice can be refrigerated and reheated in microwave (e.g., 1/2 cup [125 mL] covered at High for 30 to 60 seconds or until hot) OR frozen and reheated (e.g., 1/2 cup [125 mL] covered at high for 1/2 to 2-1/2 minutes or until hot, stirring once).

Meat, Fish, Poultry: muscle meals

Presto Pesto Lamb

In this unusual flavor combination, lamb takes on a splendid Italian character when partnered with pesto. Lamb is a rosé rather than a red meat and has no marbling in the loin. Enjoy the flavor without the fat.

Makes 2 servings

1 Serving:
Protein 27 grams
Fat 9 grams
Carbohydrate 3 grams
Calories 201

3 tbsp.	Light Pesto Sauce (page 212)	50 mL
2 tbsp.	chicken stock	25 mL
1 tbsp.	2% plain yogurt	15 mL
4	lean loin chops (about 1 lb/500 g)	4
	fresh basil, mint, coriander (cilantro) or parsley sprigs for garnish	

Method
1. In a small bowl, combine pesto, chicken stock and yogurt; set aside or chill until serving time.
2. Trim fat from chops and broil, grill or cook in non-stick pan until desired degree of doneness, about 2½ to 3 minutes per side for medium.
3. Divide sauce evenly between two plates and place chops on top.
4. Garnish with fresh basil, mint, coriander or parsley.

First cousin to the onion, garlic has been cultivated since Biblical times. Garlic is touted not only for its culinary and gastronomic qualities, but also for its health and medicinal virtues. The pungency of garlic varies with how finely it is cut and how long it is cooked.

Lamb Tandoori

2 tsp.	coriander seeds	10 mL
1 tsp.	mustard seeds	5 mL
1 tsp.	black peppercorns	5 mL
¼ cup	2% plain yogurt	50 mL
3	cloves garlic, sliced	3
1	1 inch (2 cm) piece fresh gingerroot, peeled and sliced	1
2 tsp.	lemon juice	10 mL
½ tsp.	ground cumin	2 mL
½ tsp.	tumeric	2 mL
½ tsp.	salt	2 mL
¼ tsp.	cayenne	1 mL
1	boneless leg of lamb, butterflied (5 to 6 lb/2.5 to 3 kg)	1

The spicy tandoori marinade makes this lamb extra tender and succulent. Serve with our cool Cucumber Raita (page 215) or zesty Apple Chutney (page 216) and basmati rice for a dinner with India-style flair.

Method

1. In a small non-stick skillet, heat coriander seeds, mustard seeds and peppercorns over high heat for a few minutes to toast, shaking the pan constantly.
2. In a blender, combine yogurt, toasted seeds, garlic and gingerroot. Process to make a paste.
3. Add lemon juice, cumin, tumeric, salt and cayenne; blend until smooth.
4. Trim excess fat and paper-like fell from lamb; place in a shallow dish.
5. Pour yogurt mixture over lamb being sure both sides are well coated.
6. Cover and refrigerate for at least 6 hours or overnight.
7. Bring to room temperature about 1 hour before cooking.
8. **Grill or broil** for about 15 to 20 minutes on each side. OR **roast** in 400°F (200°C) oven for 30 to 35 minutes or until meat thermometer registers 130°F (55°C) for medium rare.
9. Let stand for 10 minutes before carving.
10. Slice in thin slices across the grain. Serve hot or cold.

Makes 6 to 8 servings

1 Serving:
Protein 26 grams
Fat 7 grams
Carbohydrate 2 grams
Calories 175

Basmati is an Indian long-grain white rice and more expensive than regular long-grain white rice. It is excellent with curries or in pilafs. It should be rinsed before cooking.

Blackened Pork Chops

Succulent and juicy inside, this Cajun specialty is pungent and racy. Traditionally, these chops are cooked on a cast-iron skillet which creates heavy smoke indoors. If your exhaust system is not up to handling a spicy, dark cloud, then grill these chops outdoors on the barbecue.

Makes 2 servings

1 Serving:
Protein 26 grams
Fat 10 grams
Calories 194

1 tbsp.	Cajun Seasoning Mix	15 mL
2	boneless pork loin chops (about 8 oz/250 g total)	2
1 tbsp.	vegetable oil	15 mL

Method

1. Put seasoning mix in a small bowl; dip both sides of chops into seasoning mix, pressing to coat well.
2. In a heavy skillet, heat oil over high heat. Add pork chops to frypan; reduce heat to medium and cook until very dark brown or blackened on outside and no longer pink inside, about 4 minutes per side for 1 inch (2.5 cm) chops.

Cajun Seasoning Mix: Mix together 2 tbsp. (25 mL) paprika, 2 tsp. (10 mL) onion powder, 1 tsp. (5 mL) black pepper, 1 tsp. (5 mL) garlic powder, 1 tsp. (5 mL) dried oregano, 1 tsp. (5 mL) dried thyme, 1 tsp. (5 mL) dry mustard, ½ to 1 tsp. (2 to 5 mL) cayenne, ½ tsp. (2 mL) salt and ½ tsp. (2 mL) ground cumin; store in an airtight jar or container for up to 3 months.

Pork with Tarragon Mustard Sauce

12 oz	pork tenderloin	375 g
1 tsp.	vegetable oil	5 mL
¼ tsp.	garlic powder	1 mL
pinch	freshly ground pepper	pinch
½ cup	half and half cream	125 mL
2 tbsp.	coarse-grained mustard	25 mL
½ tsp.	dried tarragon	2 mL

Method

1. Trim off any fat from pork and rub with oil.
2. Sprinkle garlic powder and pepper over pork.
3. Grill or broil for 20 to 25 minutes or until no longer pink inside, turning once.
4. Meanwhile, in a small saucepan, bring cream to a boil; reduce heat to medium-low.
5. Stir in mustard and tarragon.
6. Simmer for 1 to 2 minutes or until slightly thickened.
7. Spoon sauce onto one side of plate.
8. Slice the tenderloin and fan slices on top of sauce.

Coarse-grained mustard gives this creamy sauce a distinctive, pleasant taste. Pork is now raised with less fat than ever before and this loin is the leanest cut on the market.

Makes 3 servings

1 Serving:
Protein 27 grams
Fat 10 grams
Carbohydrate 2 grams
Calories 206

Prepared mustards, made from ground mustard seeds, have liquids such as wine, beer, vinegar or water blended into them. Seasonings can make some mustards hot and some mild.

Flank Steak Teriyaki

A gingery Oriental marinade tenderizes this ultra-lean cut of beef. An excellent, economical dish to prepare ahead and then broil to perfection minutes before serving.

Makes 4 servings

1 Serving:
Protein 27 grams
Fat 5 grams
Carbohydrate 4 grams
Calories 169

3 tbsp.	unsweetened pineapple juice or orange juice	50 mL
2 tbsp.	soy sauce	25 mL
1 tbsp.	cider or malt vinegar	15 mL
2 tsp.	minced gingerroot	10 mL
2 tsp.	vegetable oil	10 mL
1 tsp.	honey	5 mL
1	clove garlic, minced	1
12 oz	beef flank steak or round steak	375 g

Method

1. In a shallow dish, mix juice, soy sauce, vinegar, gingerroot, oil, honey and garlic.
2. Trim excess fat from steak; score one side in crisscross cuts about 2 inches (5 cm) apart.
3. Place in the marinade, turning over to coat well. Marinate at room temperature for 30 minutes or refrigerate overnight.
4. Remove from marinade and broil or grill 4 to 6 inches (10 to 15 cm) away from heat for 4 to 5 minutes each side or until cooked to desired doneness; brush with marinade during cooking.
5. Let stand for 5 minutes and then slice thinly across the grain diagonally.

The most ancient ski in existence was found nicely preserved in a peat bog at Hoting, Sweden, dating from 2500 B.C. Scandinavian sagas feature gods of skiing.

Thai Beef Salad

5 oz	cooked lean beef	166 g
⅓ cup	lime juice	75 mL
1 tbsp.	minced fresh coriander (cilantro)	15 mL
1 tbsp.	brown sugar	15 mL
1 tbsp.	soy sauce	15 mL
2 tsp.	minced gingerroot	10 mL
¼ tsp.	grated lime zest	2 mL
pinch to ⅛ tsp.	crushed chili peppers	0.5 mL
2	green onions, trimmed and sliced into long thin strips	2
1 cup	bean sprouts	250 mL
½ cup	julienned snow peas	125 mL
½ cup	julienned sweet yellow, orange or red pepper	125 mL
½ cup	julienned English cucumber	125 mL
⅓ cup	thinly sliced red onion	75 mL
2 tbsp.	coarsely chopped unsalted peanuts fresh coriander (cilantro) sprigs for garnish	25 mL

As exotic as its name, this main course is a magnificent combination of a splendid variety of crisp, colorful vegetables, lean beef and East Asian seasonings.

Method

1. Slice beef into ¼ inch (1 cm) slices and then cut into long narrow strips.
2. In a small shallow dish, mix lime juice, coriander, sugar, soy sauce, ginger, lime zest and chili peppers; add beef strips to mixture; cover and marinate for at least 2 hours or overnight in refrigerator.
3. In a large bowl, combine green onions, bean sprouts, snow peas, peppers, cucumber and onion; add beef and marinade to vegetables.
4. Toss to coat. Sprinkle peanuts over and garnish with coriander.

Makes 2 servings

1 Serving:
Protein 29 grams
Fat 7 grams
Carbohydrate 20 grams
Calories 259

Lean and Healthy Beef Burgers

An updated version of everyone's basic favorite. Jazz up these burgers with a topping of pesto or salsa.

10 oz	lean ground beef	330 g
⅓ cup	soft whole wheat bread crumbs	75 mL
1	egg, beaten	1
1	clove garlic, minced	1
1 tbsp.	coarse-grained mustard	15 mL
¼ tsp.	freshly ground pepper	1 mL

Method

1. In a medium bowl, combine beef, bread crumbs, egg, garlic, mustard and pepper.
2. Shape into 4 patties.
3. Grill, broil or cook in non-stick skillet for 4 to 5 minutes on each side or until desired doneness.

Makes 4 patties

Tuck Into:
Flour Tortillas
Whole Wheat Pitas
Onion Buns
Toasted French Bread
Granary Buns

1 Patty:
Protein 19 grams
Fat 11 grams
Carbohydrate 6 grams
Calories 199

For Truly Sensational Burgers, top with:

Santa Fe Salsa (page 213)

Coriander Pesto (page 212)

Pepperonata (page 217)

Tahini Sauce (page 171)

Sauce Rouille (page 216)

Red Onion Rings

Part-Skim Mozzarella Cheese

Lettuce

Tomato Slices

Alfalfa Sprouts

Lemon Chicken Stir-Fry (page 195)
Flank Steak Teriyaki (page 190)

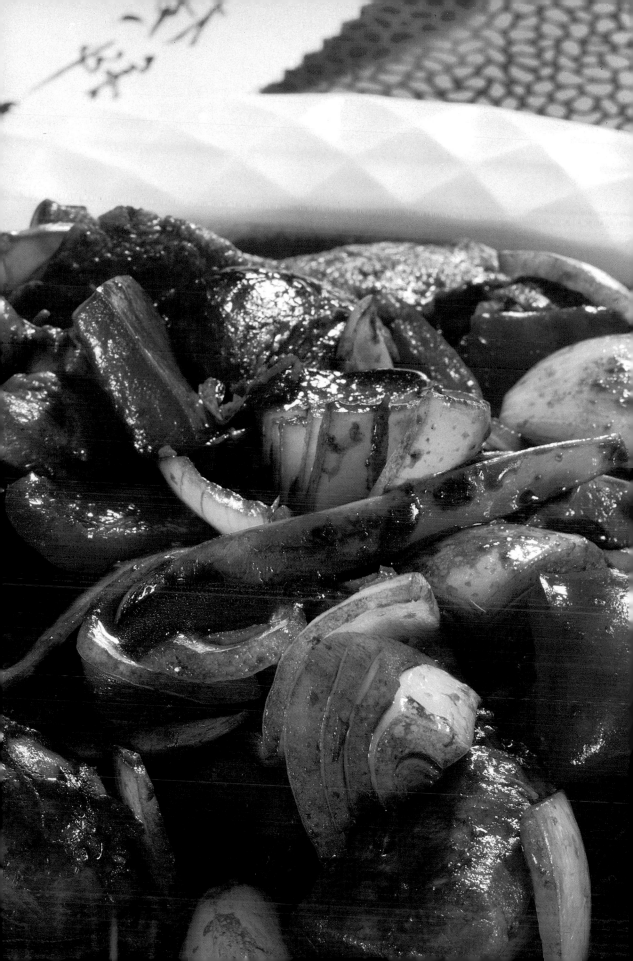

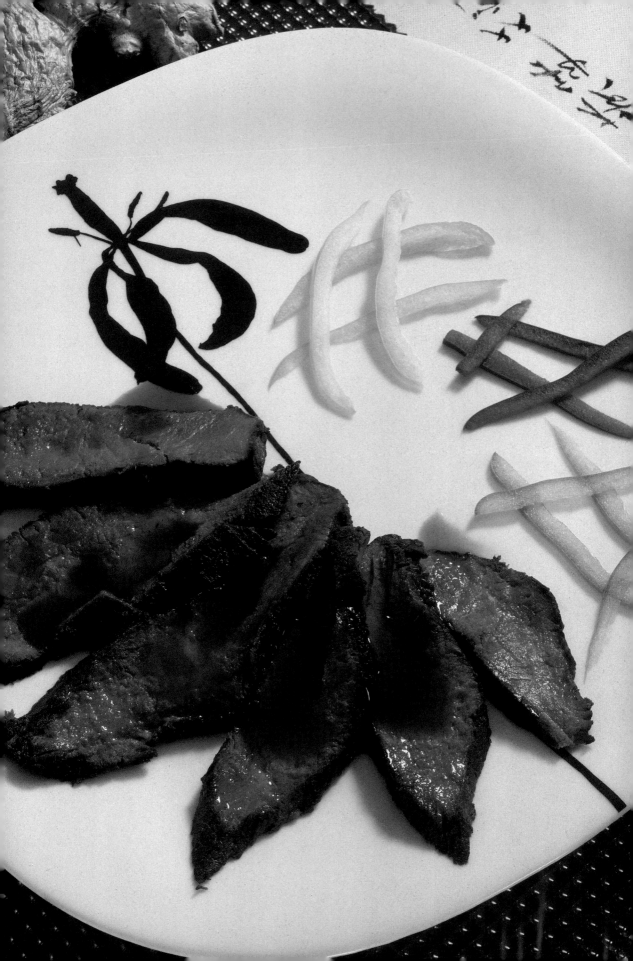

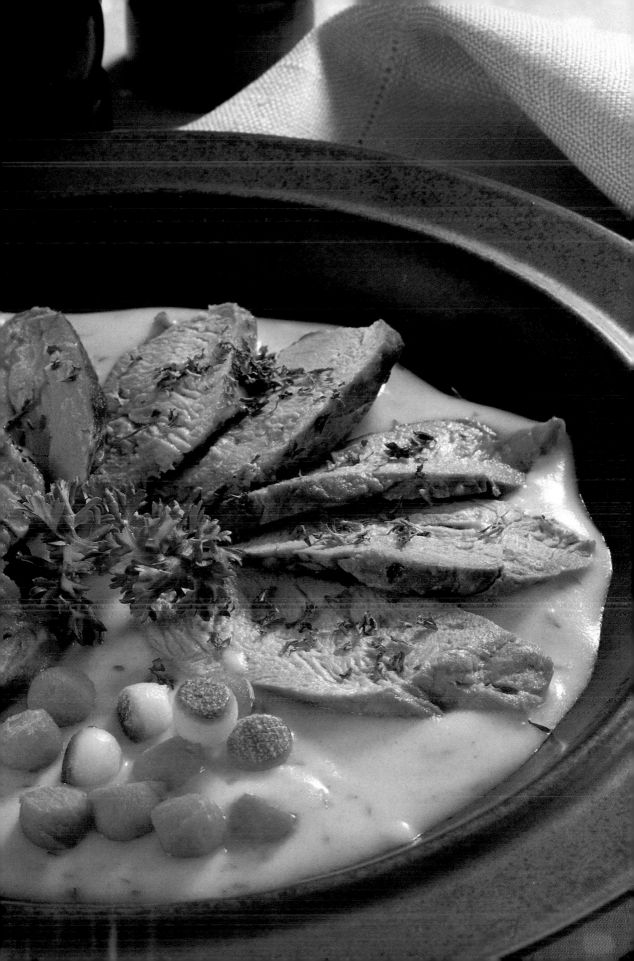

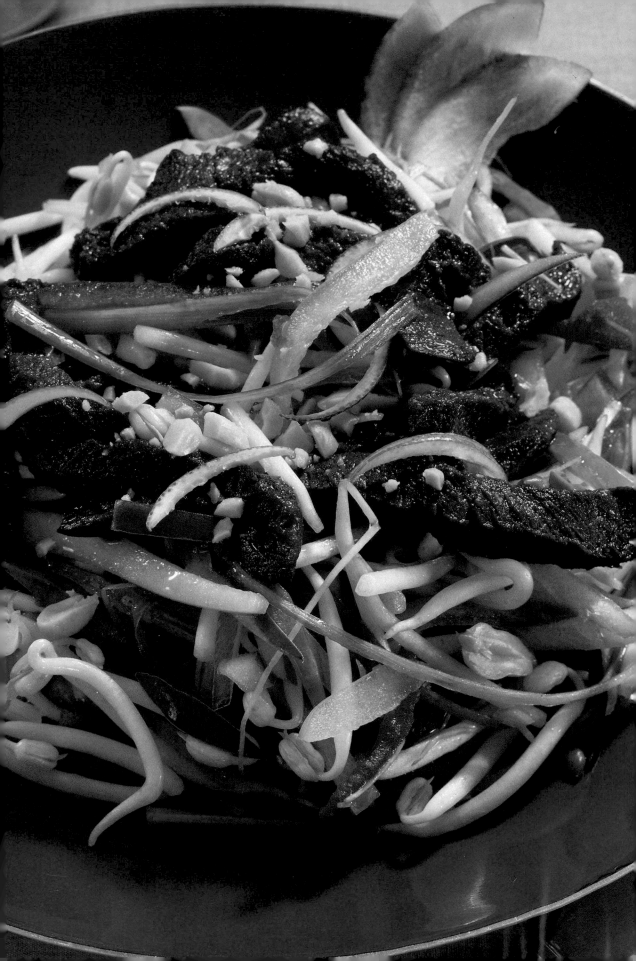

Beef and Broccoli Stir-Fry

1 tbsp.	sherry or sake	15 mL
1 tbsp.	vinegar	15 mL
1 tbsp.	soy sauce	15 mL
1 tbsp.	cornstarch	15 mL
2	broccoli stalks, including florets	2
1 tbsp.	vegetable oil	15 mL
5 oz	beef sirloin or round steak, well trimmed and sliced in long thin strips	166 g
1	onion, peeled and cut in wedges	1
1	clove garlic, minced	1
1 cup	beef stock	250 mL
2 tbsp.	julienned gingerroot	25 mL
1	10 oz (284 mL) can bamboo shoots, drained and cut in narrow strips	1

One of the brassica group unites with lean beef in an aromatic blend of ginger and soy sauce for the penultimate stir-fry. If you aren't addicted to Oriental cuisine already, after sampling this medley you'll be hooked for life.

Method

1. In a small bowl, mix sherry, vinegar, soy sauce and cornstarch.
2. Separate broccoli into florets; peel stem and slice.
3. In a wok or large non-stick skillet, heat oil over medium-high heat. Add beef strips; stir-fry for 3 to 4 minutes.
4. Add onion and garlic; stir-fry for about 3 to 4 minutes or until onion starts to soften.
5. Add broccoli, beef stock and ginger; bring to boil.
6. Cover and cook until broccoli is tender-crisp, about 2 to 3 minutes.
7. Stir in bamboo shoots; push vegetables to outside edge of pan and stir in well-mixed cornstarch mixture.
8. Cook for about 1 minute or until thickened, stirring constantly.

Makes 2 to 3 servings

1 Serving:
Protein 18 grams
Fat 7 grams
Carbohydrate 11 grams
Calories 179

Pork with Tarragon Mustard Sauce (page 189)
Thai Beef Salad (page 191)

Short-Cut Chili

Any chef can whip up this savory stew in less time than it takes to power walk three miles. Serve on rice or pasta for a complex carbohydrate boost.

1 tbsp.	olive oil	15 mL
1 lb	raw ground turkey*	500 g
1 cup	chopped onion	250 mL
1	clove garlic, minced	1
1	19 oz (540 mL) can pinto or kidney beans, undrained	1
1	19 oz (540 mL) can tomatoes, broken up	1
½ cup	water	125 mL
5 tbsp.	tomato paste	75 mL
3 tbsp.	chili powder	50 mL
2 tsp.	dried oregano	10 mL
½ tsp.	ground cumin	2 mL
½ tsp.	salt	2 mL
	2% plain yogurt for garnish	

Method

1. In a large non-stick saucepan, heat olive oil over medium heat. Add turkey, onion and garlic; cook for 5 to 10 minutes, until turkey is browned, stirring often.
2. Stir in beans with liquid, tomatoes, water, tomato paste, chili powder, oregano, cumin and salt; simmer uncovered for 10 to 15 minutes or until slightly thickened, stirring occasionally.
3. Serve in bowls garnished with yogurt, if using.

Makes 4 servings

1 Serving:
Protein 34 grams
Fat 9 grams
Carbohydrate 35 grams
Calories 357

Tip
*Ground turkey can be purchased in the refrigerated or frozen food sections of many supermarkets. You can make your own by processing boneless turkey breasts, in batches, using on/off motion until coarsely ground.

The earliest skates were made from animal bones, such as those found in France, and are thought to be 20,000 years old. The first reference to skating is in early Norse literature, around 200 B.C., but the earliest report of skating as a pastime or sport is in a British chronicle of 1180.

Lemon Chicken Stir-Fry

8 oz	boneless, skinless chicken breast	250 g
¼ cup	water	50 mL
3 tbsp.	lemon juice	50 mL
2 tsp.	soy sauce	10 mL
1 tsp.	minced gingerroot	5 mL
1 tsp.	grated lemon rind	5 mL
1 tsp.	granulated sugar	5 mL
1 tsp.	cornstarch	5 mL
1 tbsp.	vegetable oil, divided	15 mL
2	green onions, cut into 2-inch (5 cm) pieces	2
1	sweet red pepper, cut into 1-inch (2.5 cm) pieces	1
½ cup	snow peas	125 mL

Lemon makes this a distinctive and interesting stir-fry. We like it best when served with brown rice.

Method

1. Cut chicken into 1 inch (2.5 cm) pieces.
2. In a small bowl, combine water, lemon juice, soy sauce, gingerroot, rind, sugar and cornstarch; mix well.
3. Add chicken and marinate at room temperature for 30 minutes.
4. In a small non-stick skillet, heat 2 tsp. (10 mL) oil over medium-high heat. Add onion, pepper and snow peas; stir-fry for 2 to 3 minutes and remove.
5. Add remaining oil and heat until hot.
6. Drain chicken, reserving marinade.
7. Add chicken to skillet; stir-fry for about 5 minutes or until no longer pink inside.
8. Return vegetables and marinade to skillet; cook for about 1 minute or until thickened, stirring constantly.

Makes 2 servings

1 Serving:
Protein 29 grams
Fat 11 grams
Carbohydrate 11 grams
Calories 259

Chicken en Papillote

Simple enough for a fast dinner yet impressive enough for entertaining the opposing side, these juicy "meals in a pouch" are sweet with apple and leeks.

2	boneless, skinless chicken breasts (about 8 oz/250 g total)	2
2 tsp.	coarse-grained mustard	10 mL
1 tbsp.	butter or soft margarine	15 mL
1 cup	sliced apple	250 mL
½ cup	sliced leeks	125 mL
½ cup	sliced mushrooms	125 mL
½ cup	grated carrot	125 mL
3 tbsp.	apple brandy, brandy or apple juice	50 mL
2 tbsp.	chopped fresh parsley	25 mL
1 tsp.	dried tarragon	5 mL
	freshly ground pepper	

Makes 2 servings

Tip
Packets can be prepared ahead of time and chilled until ready to cook.

1 Serving:
Protein 29 grams
Fat 9 grams
Carbohydrate 10 grams
Calories 237

Method

1. Cut two sheets 12 x 13 inches (30 x 32 cm) of parchment paper. (If cooking in a conventional oven, foil can be substituted.)
2. Fold in half lengthwise, crease. Open each one and place a chicken breast half on each in the middle near the crease. Spread mustard on chicken.
3. In a small non-stick skillet, heat butter over medium heat. Add apple, leeks, mushrooms and carrots. Sauté for 1 to 2 minutes or until softened; stir in brandy (if using), parsley, tarragon and pepper to taste.
4. Spoon vegetable mixture including liquids over chicken.
5. Fold top half of paper over vegetables; seal well by making a double ½ inch (1 cm) fold on all open edges.
6. **Microwave** at High for 3 to 4 minutes or until chicken is no longer pink. Let stand for 5 minutes. OR **bake** on baking sheet in 400°F (200°C) oven for about 15 to 20 minutes or until chicken is no longer pink.
7. Place each package on serving plate and open just before eating.

Turkey Paupiettes

4	skinless turkey cutlets (about 1 lb/500 g total)	4
8 oz	fresh spinach	250 g
2 tbsp.	olive oil, divided	25 mL
¼ cup	finely chopped onion	50 mL
1	clove garlic, minced	1
1	egg, well beaten	1
¼ cup	fine dry bread crumbs	50 mL
2 tsp.	lemon juice	10 mL
½ tsp.	nutmeg	2 mL
¼ tsp.	pepper	1 mL
¼ tsp.	salt	1 mL

Nice as a change from ordinary beef or poultry, these colorful rolls combine an iron-rich vegetable and a low fat meat. For a company menu, serve with Lemon Rice Pilaf (page 162) and our Watercress and Beets Vinaigrette (page 116).

Method

1. Pound turkey cutlets to ¼ inch (0.5 cm) thickness.
2. Remove tough stems of spinach and rinse well.
3. With just the water clinging to the leaves, cook spinach, covered, for 3 minutes or until tender.
4. Drain well, pressing out moisture, and chop finely.
5. Heat 1 tsp. (5 mL) of the oil in a non-stick skillet. Add onion and garlic; sauté for 2 to 3 minutes or until onion is limp.
6. Remove from heat and stir in spinach, egg, bread crumbs, lemon juice, nutmeg, pepper and salt.
7. Spoon ¼ of spinach mixture onto one end of each turkey cutlet.
8. Roll turkey around spinach securing ends and edges with toothpicks.
9. Wipe out skillet with paper towel, add remaining oil and heat over medium heat. Add turkey and cook for about 15 to 18 minutes or until turkey is no longer pink inside, turning frequently.
10. Let sit for 5 minutes and then cut each roll into thick slices.

Makes 4 servings

1 Serving:
Protein 30 grams
Fat 10 grams
Carbohydrate 7 grams
Calories 238

Rosemary Grilled Chicken

Barbecued chicken is subtly enhanced by the fresh rosemary in this effortless yet elegant recipe. Skinless poultry is an excellent source of low-fat protein.

Makes 2 servings

1 Serving:
Protein 28 grams
Fat 8 grams
Calories 184

2	boneless, skinless chicken breasts (about 8 oz/250 g total)	2
1 tbsp.	fresh rosemary OR 1 tsp. (5 mL) dried	15 mL
1 tbsp.	olive oil	15 mL
1 tbsp.	raspberry vinegar	15 mL
1 tsp.	Dijon mustard	5 mL

Method

1. Pat rosemary onto both sides of chicken.
2. In a small shallow dish, mix oil, vinegar and mustard together.
3. Add chicken; marinate for ½ to 2 hours in refrigerator turning once or twice to coat both sides.
4. Grill or broil for about 4 minutes per side or until no longer pink inside.
5. Slice each breast into about 4 slices and fan out on plate.

Diablo Grilled Chicken

2 tbsp.	lime juice	25 mL
1 tbsp.	olive oil	15 mL
1	clove garlic, minced	1
⅛ to ¼ tsp.	coarsely crushed black peppercorns or chili peppers	0.5 to 1 mL
4	boneless, skinless chicken breasts (about 1 lb/500 g total) lime wedges for garnish	4

Wicked and wonderful, these lively seasonings transform chicken into a delectable dish. Top with Santa Fe Salsa (page 213) for added gusto.

Method
1. In a shallow dish, mix lime juice, oil, garlic and pepper; add chicken and marinate for ½ hour or up to 8 hours in the refrigerator.
2. Broil or grill or cook in small non-stick skillet for 4 to 5 minutes per side or until no longer pink inside.
3. Garnish with lime wedges.

Makes 4 servings

1 Serving:
Protein 28 grams
Fat 8 grams
Calories 184

Accompaniment
Dilled Bean and Carrot Packets: On a large piece of heavy-duty foil, combine 1 cup (250 mL) halved green or yellow beans, 1 cup (250 mL) whole baby carrots, ½ cup (125 mL) sliced onions, 2 tsp. (10 mL) olive oil, 1 tbsp. (15 mL) chopped fresh dill (¼ tsp./2 mL dried) and freshly ground pepper to taste. Toss to mix well; fold and seal open edges with a double fold. Cook on barbecue grill about 4 inches (10 cm) above heat for 20 to 30 minutes or in 350°F (180°C) oven for 20 to 30 minutes or until tender-crisp. (Time will vary with freshness of vegetables and heat of fire.) Serve plain or drizzle with ¼ cup (50 mL) light sour cream mixed with ½ tsp. (2 mL) lemon juice.

Turkey Paillards

These super lean cutlets are simply and quickly sautéed before serving with a mango sauce redolent of mint and tart with yogurt and lime.

Makes 2 servings

1 Serving:
Protein 28 grams
Fat 10 grams
Calories 202

8 oz	skinless turkey cutlets	250 g
2 tsp.	vegetable oil	10 mL
2 tsp.	lime juice	10 mL
½ cup	Mango Mint Sauce	125 mL

Method

1. Pound turkey cutlets to ½ inch (1 cm) thickness.
2. In a non-stick skillet, heat oil over medium heat; add turkey and cook for about 2 minutes on each side or until golden brown and no longer pink inside.
3. Squeeze lime juice over cutlets.
4. Serve with Mango Mint Sauce.

Mango Mint Sauce: In a small bowl combine 1 cup (250 mL) diced, peeled mango or peaches, ⅓ cup (75 mL) 2% plain yogurt and 2 tbsp. (25 mL) coarsely chopped mint. Cover and refrigerate for at least 2 hours to blend flavors.

Two Americans developed figure skating into an art. E. W. Bushnell invented steel blades in 1848, providing the precision skate needed for more intricate figures, and the first innovator and teacher was Jackson Haines, a ballet instructor.

Fish and Veggies in a Packet

2	sole or orange roughy fillets (about 12 oz/375 g total)	2	
1 tbsp.	lemon juice	15 mL	
¼ cup	chicken stock	50 mL	
½ cup	julienned sweet red or yellow pepper	125 mL	
¼ cup	julienned zucchini	125 mL	
½ cup	julienned green onions	125 mL	
¼ cup	chopped fresh dill	50 mL	
⅛ tsp.	salt	0.5 mL	
	freshly ground pepper		

A colorful "package" fixed with no fuss and little mess. Just add a baked potato for a meal of mellow flavors and almost no fat.

Method

1. Cut 2 sheets 12 inch (30 cm) square of parchment paper. (If cooking in conventional oven, aluminum foil can be substituted.)
2. Fold in half diagonally and crease. Open each square and place a fish fillet on one half near the crease.
3. Drizzle lemon juice over each fillet.
4. In a small skillet, heat chicken stock; add peppers, zucchini and green onions. Simmer, stirring often, for 2 to 3 minutes or until softened.
5. Stir in dill, salt and pepper to taste.
6. Spoon vegetable mixture including liquid evenly over fish fillets.
7. Fold top half of paper over vegetables; seal well by making a double ½ inch (1 cm) fold on all open edges.
8. **Microwave** at High for 3½ to 4½ minutes or until flesh is opaque. Let stand for 5 minutes. OR **bake** on baking sheet in 400°F (200°C) oven for 7 to 10 minutes or until flesh is opaque.
9. Place each package on serving plate and open or slash just before eating. Pockets can be prepared ahead of time and chilled until ready to cook.

Makes 2 servings

1 Serving:
Protein 26 grams
Fat 2 grams
Carbohydrate 6 grams
Calories 146

Mediterranean Sea Bass

Tender sea bass is made exotic and savory in this Mediterranean-inspired recipe. Serve with couscous and a deep green vegetable for a winning dinner combo.

2	sea bass fillets or any other firm fish, skin removed (about 1 lb/500 g)	2
1 tbsp.	honey	15 mL
2 tsp.	lemon juice	10 mL
2 tbsp.	olive oil	25 mL
1 tsp.	cumin	5 mL
1 tsp.	paprika	5 mL
½ tsp.	cinnamon	2 mL
¾ tsp.	salt	4 mL
½ tsp.	pepper	2 mL
pinch	cayenne	pinch
2	cloves garlic, minced	2
¼ cup	freshly chopped coriander (cilantro) leaves or parsley	50 mL

Serves 2 to 3

1 Serving:
Protein 28 grams
Fat 11 grams
Carbohydrate 6 grams
Calories 235

Method

1. Preheat oven to 400°F (200°C).
2. In small bowl, whisk together honey, lemon juice, 1 tbsp. of the oil, cumin, paprika, cinnamon, salt, pepper, cayenne, garlic and coriander.
3. Spread spice mixture over fish fillets. Cover and refrigerate for about 1 hour.
4. Heat remaining oil in a non-stick skillet over high heat. Cook sea bass for 2 minutes, turning once.
5. Transfer to foil-lined baking sheet and bake until fish flakes easily when tested with a fork, about 10 minutes.

Quick 'n' Easy Herbed Fish Fillets

½ cup	fine dry bread crumbs	125 mL
1 tsp.	dried dillweed or tarragon	5 mL
¼ tsp.	salt	1 mL
pinch	freshly ground pepper	pinch
½ cup	2% plain yogurt	125 mL
2	haddock or cod fillets, fresh or frozen and thawed (about 8 oz/250 g total)	2

Method

1. In a shallow dish or plate, combine bread crumbs, dill, salt and pepper.
2. Put yogurt in another shallow dish.
3. Dip both sides of fish fillets in yogurt and then in crumb mixture; pat crumbs onto fish to cover well.
4. Place on non-stick baking sheet.
5. Bake in 425°F (220°C) oven for 5 minutes; turn and cook for about 5 minutes longer until crust is browned and flesh is opaque.

Variation

Substitute sole, orange roughy, Boston bluefish or perch for the haddock or cod in this recipe.

This homemade version of commercial fish sticks has a nicely seasoned crisp crust highlighted with dill. Delicious when served with Sauce Piquante (page 214) and Lemon Rice Pilaf (page 162).

Makes 2 servings

1 Serving:
Protein 22 grams
Fat 2 grams
Carbohydrate 14 grams
Calories 162

Bouillabaisse with Soul

Stunning, sexy, rich with saffron and fennel, this fish soup from Marseilles would please King Neptune himself. The Rouille, with its robust garlic and pepper flavors, is a "must" when serving.

2 tsp.	olive oil	10 mL
½ cup	chopped onion	125 mL
½ cup	chopped celery	125 mL
¼ cup	finely diced carrot	50 mL
1	19 oz (540 mL) can tomatoes, broken up	1
2 cups	chicken stock	500 mL
¾ cup	dry white wine	175 mL
½ cup	chopped green pepper	125 mL
1 tsp.	dried thyme	5 mL
½ tsp.	fennel seeds	2 mL
⅛ tsp.	saffron threads OR pinch of saffron powder	0.5 mL
1	bay leaf	1
	freshly ground pepper	
8 oz	white fish fillets, cut in bite-sized pieces (e.g., cod, halibut, sole or monkfish)	250 g
8 oz	mussels, scrubbed and debearded	250 g
½ cup	Rouille Sauce (page 216)	125 mL

Makes 2 to 3 servings

1 Serving:
Protein 14 grams
Fat 6 grams
Carbohydrate 13 grams
Calories 162

Method

1. In a large saucepan, heat oil over medium heat. Add onion, celery and carrot; sauté for about 5 minutes or until vegetables have softened; add tomatoes, stock, white wine, green pepper, thyme, fennel, saffron, bay leaf and pepper to taste.
2. Cover and bring to boil; reduce heat and simmer for 20 to 30 minutes or until vegetables are tender. (Recipe can be prepared ahead to this point. Cover and refrigerate for up to 2 days. Reheat before continuing.)
3. Just before serving, add fish pieces and mussels; cover and cook for about 5 minutes or until flesh is opaque and mussels have opened.
4. Discard bay leaf and any mussels that have not opened.
5. Serve in soup bowls topped with a spoonful of Rouille Sauce.

Racquetball was invented by Joe Sobek at the Greenwich, Connecticut, YMCA in the early 1960s.

New England Fish Chowder

2 tsp.	butter or soft margarine	10 mL
½ cup	chopped onion	125 mL
⅔ cup	chopped celery, including leaves	150 mL
1 cup	chicken stock	250 mL
1	large potato, peeled and finely diced	1
¼ tsp.	dried thyme	1 mL
⅛ tsp.	salt	0.5 mL
	freshly ground white pepper	
1 tsp.	Worcestershire sauce	5 mL
⅔ cup	2% evaporated milk	150 mL
⅔ cup	2% milk	150 mL
5 oz	cod, haddock or Boston bluefish fillets, fresh or frozen and thawed, cut in bite-sized pieces	166 g
	chopped parsley for garnish	

Method

1. In a medium non-stick saucepan, melt butter over medium heat. Add onion and celery; sauté for 3 to 4 minutes or until vegetables have softened.
2. Add stock, potatoes, thyme, salt and pepper to taste; cover and bring to boil.
3. Cook for about 10 minutes or until potatoes are almost tender.
4. Add Worcestershire sauce, evaporated milk, 2% milk and fish pieces; cover and cook for about 5 minutes or until flesh is opaque.
5. Sprinkle each bowl with minced parsley if using.

Makes 2 to 3 servings

1 Serving:
Protein 17 grams
Fat 5 grams
Carbohydrate 22 grams
Calories 201

Monkfish Brochette

Firm-fleshed monkfish is ideally suited for this citrus marinade and grilling. If using wooden skewers, soak in water for 30 minutes before threading to prevent scorching.

2 tbsp.	orange juice	25 mL
1 tbsp.	dry white wine or vermouth	15 mL
1 tbsp.	olive oil	15 mL
1 tbsp.	minced fresh parsley	15 mL
1 tsp.	grated orange rind	5 mL
1 tsp.	lemon juice	5 mL
1 tsp.	dried oregano	5 mL
1	clove garlic, minced	1
pinch	salt	pinch
	freshly ground pepper	
8 oz	monkfish, cut into 1-inch (2.5 cm) cubes	250 g

Makes 2 servings

1 Serving:
Protein 24 grams
Fat 12 grams
Carbohydrate 1 gram
Calories 208

Method

1. In a shallow dish, mix orange juice, wine, oil, parsley, orange rind, lemon juice, oregano, garlic, salt and pepper to taste; add fish.
2. Toss to coat well; marinate for at least 2 hours or up to 8 hours in refrigerator.
3. Thread fish on skewers.
4. Broil or grill about 4 inches (10 cm) from heat for about 5 minutes on each side or until flesh is opaque, brushing with marinade during cooking.
5. Serve any extra marinade as a sauce to spoon over fish.

Blackened Red Snapper

5 tsp.	Cajun Seasoning Mix (page 188)	25 mL
2	red snapper or catfish fillets (about 8 oz/250 g total)	2
1 tbsp.	vegetable oil	15 mL

Method

1. Spread seasoning mix on a flat plate; dip both sides of fillets into seasoning mix, pressing to coat well.
2. In a heavy skillet (preferably cast iron), heat oil over high heat; add fillets; reduce heat to medium and **cook** for 2 to 2½ minutes on each side or until flesh is opaque. OR **grill** on greased grill about 4 inches (10 cm) above heat for 2 to 2½ minutes per side or until flesh is opaque.

Microwave Version

Coat fillets as directed in recipe. Arrange in microwaveable baking dish; cover with wax paper. Microwave at High for 3 to 4 minutes or until flesh is opaque.

Rosy-hued, titillating to the palate, the fish in this recipe is easy to prepare and trendy to serve. Grill outside for quick cleanup and a kitchen free of smoke.

Makes 2 servings

1 Serving:
Protein 24 grams
Fat 9 grams
Calories 177

Mighty Mussels

For a classy "cheap and cheerful" appetizer this is it. Low in calories and fat, these mussels should be served in large bowls with plenty of crusty bread for sopping up the fragrant juices.

Makes 2 appetizer servings

1 Serving
Protein 7 grams
Fat 3 grams
Carbohydrate 1.5 grams
Calories 61

Tip
Mussels are best in fall and winter. Check to make sure the nearly smooth blue/black shells are shut tight. To determine if a mussel is still alive, hold it between thumb and forefinger and try to slide the upper and lower shells across one another. A fresh mussel will not slide.

1 lb	mussels (about 12)	500 g
¼ cup	dry white wine	50 mL
2 tbsp.	minced shallots	25 mL
1 tbsp.	minced fresh parsley	15 mL
1 tsp.	olive oil	5 mL
1 to 2	cloves garlic, minced	1 to 2
¼ tsp.	dried thyme	1 mL
	freshly ground pepper	
	lemon wedges for garnish	

Method
1. With a stiff brush scrub mussels under cold running water; discard ones that are open. Pull off beards.
2. In a large saucepan, combine mussels, wine, shallots, parsley, oil, garlic, thyme and pepper to taste.
3. Cover and bring to boil.
4. Cook for about 5 minutes or until mussel shells open.
5. Any closed mussels should be discarded.
6. Pass lemon wedges to squeeze on at serving time.

Falafel (page 171)
Kiwi Sorbet (page 228)

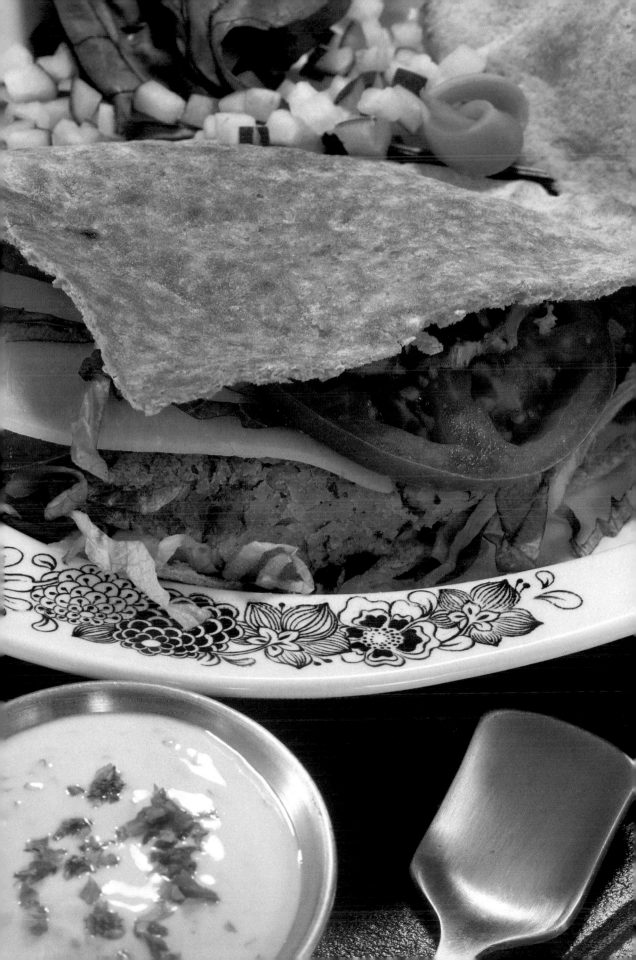

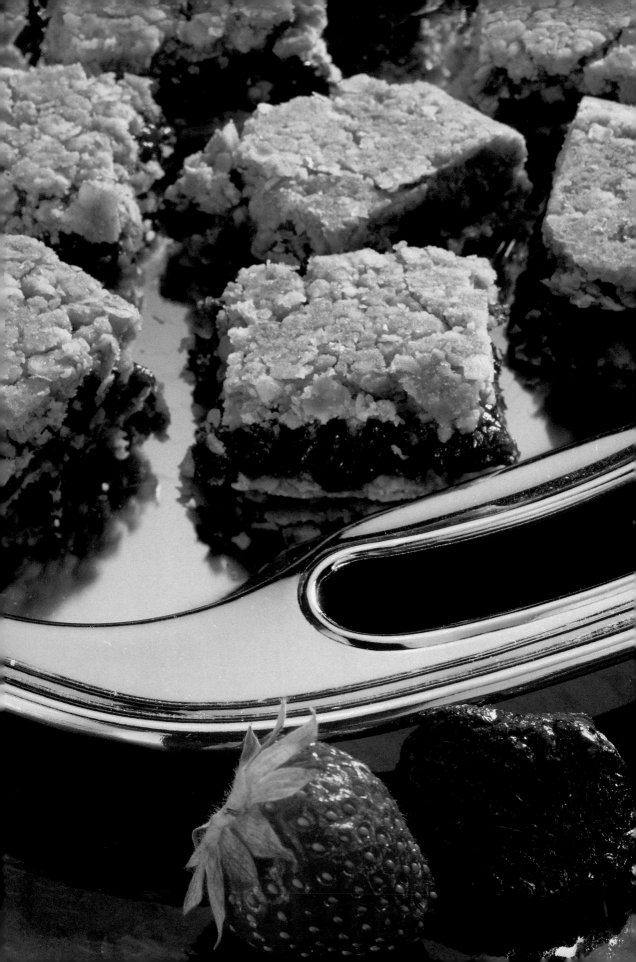

Grilled Swordfish Steaks

2 tbsp.	lime juice	25 mL
1 tbsp.	olive oil	15 mL
1 tsp.	fresh rosemary OR ¼ tsp. (1 mL) dried	5 mL
1 tsp.	fresh thyme OR ¼ tsp. (1 mL) dried	5 mL
¼ tsp.	fennel or anise seeds	1 mL
2	swordfish steaks (about 12 oz/ 375 g total)	2
	fresh rosemary sprigs and lime wedges for garnish	

Method

1. In a shallow dish, combine lime juice, oil, rosemary, thyme and fennel seeds; add swordfish and marinate at room temperature for 30 minutes, turning fish over once or twice to coat both sides.
2. Grill or broil for about 4 minutes per side or until flesh is opaque and firm to the touch.
3. Garnish with rosemary sprigs and lime.

Accompaniment

Herb and Garlic Potato Packets: Scrub 6 small new potatoes (or 3 larger potatoes quartered) and pat dry with paper towels. On a large piece of heavy-duty foil, toss potatoes with 1 tbsp. (15 mL) olive oil, 2 minced garlic cloves, 1 tsp. (5 mL) fresh oregano or thyme, ½ tsp. (2 mL) grated lemon rind and pepper to taste. Bring edges of foil together; pleat to seal. Barbecue for 30 to 40 minutes or until potatoes are tender. Alternatively, bake in 350°F (180°C) oven for 30 to 40 minutes.

A meaty fish that marries well with herbs from Provence and is superb grilled. Serve with Light Pesto (page 212) or Santa Fe Salsa (page 213) for a menu in vogue. Fish is low in fat and should be incorporated into our diets at least three times a week.

Makes 2 servings

1 Serving:
Protein 17 grams
Fat 11 grams
Carbohydrate 1 gram
Calories 171

Orange Poached Pears (page 221)
Oat Squares (page 223)

Salmon Steaks au Poivre

This is a wonderful change of pace from the original beef version. Better yet, salmon is absolutely loaded with omega-3-fatty acids which may be a boon for your arteries.

1 tsp.	minced thyme, OR ¼ tsp. (1 mL) dried	5 mL
1 tsp.	coarsely crushed black peppercorns	5 mL
2	salmon steaks (about 12 oz/ 375 g total)	2
1 tbsp.	olive oil	15 mL
1 tbsp.	lemon juice	15 mL
	fresh thyme sprigs for garnish	
	lemon wedges for garnish	

Makes 2 servings

1 Serving:
Protein 40 grams
Fat 18 grams
Calories 322

Method
1. Pat thyme and pepper on both sides of salmon.
2. In a shallow dish, mix oil and lemon juice; add salmon.
3. Marinate at room temperature for 30 minutes, turning once or twice to coat both sides.
4. Grill, broil or cook in non-stick pan for about 4 minutes per side or until flesh is opaque.
5. Garnish with thyme sprigs and lemon wedges.

Marinated Dill Trout

A savory marinade and the delicacy of trout meld into a glorious fish dish. Prepare the fillet while cooking a barley or rice pilaf for a totally satisfying meal.

1 tbsp.	lemon juice	15 mL
1 tbsp.	chopped fresh dill	15 mL
1 tsp.	Dijon mustard	5 mL
1	6 oz (180 g) trout fillet	1

Makes 1 serving

1 Serving:
Protein 38 grams
Fat 19 grams
Calories 323

Method
1. In a shallow dish, combine lemon juice, dill and mustard; add trout, turning over to coat both sides and marinate for 30 minutes at room temperature.
2. Remove from marinade and **broil, grill or cook** in non-stick pan for 4 to 5 minutes or until flesh is opaque. OR **microwave** at High for 1½ to 2 minutes; let stand for 2 minutes.
3. Serve any extra marinade as a sauce.

West Coast Shrimp

8 oz	cooked shrimp	250 g
½	lemon, thinly sliced	½
½	medium onion, thinly sliced	½
2 tbsp.	cider vinegar	25 mL
1 tbsp.	vegetable oil	15 mL
1 tbsp.	lemon or lime juice	15 mL
1 tsp.	granulated sugar	5 mL
⅛ tsp.	salt	0.5 mL
1	small clove garlic, minced	1
⅛ tsp.	dry mustard	0.5 mL
pinch	crushed chili peppers	pinch
	freshly ground pepper	
	lettuce leaves for garnish	
	parsley sprigs for garnish	

Fresh and lively flavors make an elegant first course or a gratifying entrée when accompanied by our Brown Rice Salad (page 119).

Method

1. In a large bowl, mix shrimp, lemon and onion together.
2. In a saucepan, combine vinegar, oil, lemon juice, sugar, salt, garlic, mustard, chili peppers and pepper to taste.
3. Bring to boil; remove from heat and cool slightly.
4. Pour over shrimp, lemon and onions.
5. Cover and refrigerate for at least 6 hours or overnight, stirring occasionally.
6. Drain off and discard marinade.
7. To serve, arrange shrimp mixture on a lettuce leaf.
8. Garnish with parsley.

Makes 4 appetizer or 2 lunch entrées

1 Main Course Serving:
Protein 24 grams
Fat 8 grams
Carbohydrate 4 grams
Calories 184

Sauces and Accompaniments:
dynamic duos

Light Pesto Sauce

The aromatic flavors of this herb mélange complement soups, bruschetta, burgers, grilled meats and pasta. Pesto means "pounded" – but a food processor replaces the original pestle and mortar in this fat-reduced adaptation.

Makes 2/3 cup (150 mL)

2 Tablespoons:
Protein 5 grams
Fat 10 grams
Carbohydrate 5 grams
Calories 130

2 cups	fresh basil, parsley, coriander (cilantro) or mint leaves, loosely packed	500 g
½ cup	Italian parsley	125 mL
¼ cup	olive oil	50 mL
2	cloves garlic, sliced	2
½ cup	grated Parmesan cheese	125 mL

Method
1. In food processor, combine basil, Italian parsley, oil, garlic and Parmesan cheese; process until finely chopped and well mixed.
2. Serve immediately or refrigerate for up to 1 week or freeze up to one month.

Serving Suggestion
Pesto pasta: Mix 3 tbsp. (50 mL) pesto sauce with 2 tbsp. (25 mL) chicken stock and 1 tbsp. (15 mL) 2% plain yogurt. Toss with 4 oz (125 g) cooked pasta. Add Parmesan cheese to taste. Makes 2 servings.

Santa Fe Salsa

1	large tomato, finely diced	1
¼ cup	finely diced onion	50 mL
1 tbsp.	finely diced pickled jalapeno peppers OR 2 tbsp. (25 mL) finely diced canned green chilies	15 mL
1 tbsp.	finely chopped coriander (cilantro) or parsley	15 mL
1 tsp.	lime juice or lemon juice	5 mL
1 tsp.	olive oil	5 mL

Method
1. In a small bowl, combine tomato, onion, peppers, coriander, lime juice and oil.
2. Serve immediately or cover and refrigerate for up to 8 hours.

A lively relish and versatile Mexican accompaniment, great with grilled meats, burgers, fish, nachos or as a dip. For breakfast with a Mexican spirit, top scrambled eggs with Santa Fe Salsa and enjoy.

Makes 1-1/4 cups (300 mL)

2 Tablespoons:
Fat 0.5 gram
Carbohydrate 1 gram
Calories 8

Dilled Cucumber Sauce

⅓ cup	grated English cucumber	75 mL
¼ cup	light mayonnaise	50 mL
¼ cup	2% plain yogurt	50 mL
2 tbsp.	sliced green onion	25 mL
1 tsp.	minced fresh dill	5 mL

Method
1. In a small bowl, combine cucumber, mayonnaise, yogurt, green onion and dill.
2. Serve immediately or cover and refrigerate for up to 8 hours.

Fresh and light, this is perfect with any variety of fish.

Makes 1/2 cup (125 mL)

2 Tablespoons:
Protein 0.5 gram
Fat 3.5 grams
Carbohydrate 1 gram
Calories 37

Basic Tomato Sauce

This rich, red sauce is a must in any repertoire of survival cooking. If you have containers of this basic sauce tucked away in your freezer, you can whip up delicious pasta dishes and pizza in no time flat.

2	28 oz (796 mL) cans tomatoes OR 6 cups (1.5 L) fresh tomatoes, peeled and chopped	2
1 cup	chopped onion	250 mL
5 tbsp.	tomato paste	65 mL
2	cloves garlic, minced	2
2 tsp.	dried oregano OR 2 tbsp. (25 mL) fresh	10 mL
1 tsp.	dried basil OR 1 tbsp. (15 mL) fresh	5 mL
1 tsp.	granulated sugar	5 mL
½ tsp.	salt	2 mL
¼ tsp.	hot red pepper sauce	1 mL

Method
1. In a large saucepan, combine tomatoes, onion, tomato paste, garlic, oregano, basil, sugar, salt and pepper sauce; mash tomatoes with potato masher or fork.
2. Bring to a boil; reduce heat and simmer uncovered for about 1 hour or until thickened. Sauce can be stored in refrigerator for up to 4 days or in freezer for up to 4 months.

Makes 4 cups (1 L)

1/2 Cup:
Protein 2 grams
Carbohydrate 10 grams
Calories 48

Sauce Piquante

Nice with veal or turkey, this sauce derives its liveliness from the capers and garlic. The lemon also makes it a good partner for fish.

2	anchovy fillets	2
2 tbsp.	olive oil	25 mL
⅓ cup	finely chopped Italian parsley	75 mL
2 tbsp.	finely chopped capers	25 mL
2 tbsp.	minced shallots	25 mL
1	clove garlic, minced	1
2 to 3 tbsp.	lemon juice	25 to 50 mL
	freshly ground pepper	

Method
1. Rinse anchovy fillets and pat dry with paper towels.
2. In a small bowl, mash anchovies and oil with a fork; mix in parsley, capers, shallots, garlic, 2 tbsp. (25 mL) lemon juice and pepper to taste.
3. Taste and increase lemon juice if desired, especially if serving with fish.

Makes 1/3 cup (75 mL)

2 Tablespoons:
Protein 1 gram
Fat 8 grams
Carbohydrate 1 gram
Calories 80

Cucumber Raita

¾ cup	grated English cucumber	175 mL
½ cup	2% plain yogurt	125 mL
2 tsp.	chopped fresh coriander (cilantro) or mint leaves	10 mL
1	clove garlic, minced	1
⅛ tsp.	ground cumin	0.5 mL
pinch	salt	pinch
	freshly ground pepper	
⅓ cup	diced tomato or red pepper (optional)	75 mL

Excellent with lamb, this is a fresh and delightful sauce.

Method

1. Combine cucumber, yogurt, coriander, garlic, cumin, salt and pepper to taste.
2. Stir in tomato, if using. Cover and refrigerate for at least 1 hour or up to 2 days.

Makes 1 cup (250 mL)

2 Tablespoons:
Protein 1 gram
Carbohydrate 2 grams
Calories 12

Indispensable Cheese Sauce

1 tbsp.	butter or soft margarine	15 mL
4 tsp.	all-purpose flour	20 mL
1⅓ cups	skim milk	325 mL
⅓ cup	grated cheddar or Parmesan cheese	75 mL
⅛ tsp.	salt	0.5 mL
pinch	nutmeg	pinch
	freshly ground pepper	

Cooked veggies, baked potatoes, even pasta take on a creamy, comforting Hollandaise-like presence without all the fat.

Microwave Method

1. In an 8 cup (2 L) microwaveable measure or bowl, microwave butter at High for 40 seconds or until melted.
2. Stir in flour; gradually stir or whisk in milk.
3. Microwave at High for 1½ minutes; stir.
4. Microwave at High for 2½ to 3½ minutes longer, stirring twice or until slightly thickened.
5. Stir in cheese, salt, nutmeg and pepper to taste.
6. Microwave at High for 40 seconds longer or until cheese has melted.

Makes about 1 cup (250 mL)

2 Tablespoons:
Protein 2 grams
Fat 2 grams
Carbohydrate 2 grams
Calories 34

Serving Suggestion

For a comfy, cozy supper for one, moisten one serving of your favorite cooked pasta with our Indispensable Cheese Sauce. Top with bread crumbs and Parmesan cheese. Bake in 350°F (180°C) oven until top is browned.

Apple Chutney

With or without mint, hot or cold, this chutney is delightful with lamb, cold meats or curries. Try it on crackers with cheese for an unusually tasty snack.

1½ cups	peeled and chopped apple	375 mL
½ cup	peeled, seeded and chopped tomato	375 mL
2 tbsp.	raisins	25 mL
2 tbsp.	cider or malt vinegar	25 mL
2 tbsp.	chopped fresh mint (optional)	25 mL
1 tbsp.	water	15 mL
1 tbsp.	brown sugar	15 mL
1 tsp.	minced gingerroot	5 mL
½ tsp.	coriander seeds	2 mL
⅛ tsp.	ground cinnamon	0.5 mL
⅛ tsp.	salt	0.5 mL
	freshly ground pepper	

**Makes 1 cup
(250 mL)**

2 Tablespoons:
Carbohydrate 7 grams
Calories 28

Method

1. In a small saucepan, combine apple, tomato, raisins, vinegar, mint if using, water, brown sugar, ginger, coriander, cinnamon, salt and pepper to taste.
2. Cover and bring to **boil**; reduce heat and simmer for about 10 minutes or until apple is tender and mixture has thickened. OR combine ingredients in 4 cup (1 L) glass measure; cover and **microwave** at High for 5 to 10 minutes or until fruit is tender and mixture has thickened.
3. Serve immediately or cover and refrigerate up to 2 weeks.

Sauce Rouille

Rich and robust to taste, this creamy, russet-colored sauce is excellent with fish, grilled meats and particularly with soups such as bouillabaisse.

½ cup	chopped green pepper	125 mL
¼ cup	water	50 mL
¼ cup	chopped canned pimento	50 mL
2 to 3 drops	hot pepper sauce	2 to 3 drops
1	clove garlic, crushed	1
1 tbsp.	olive oil	15 mL
1 tbsp.	fine dry bread crumbs	15 mL

**Makes 1/2 cup
(125 mL)**

2 Tablespoons:
Fat 3 grams
Carbohydrate 3 grams
Calories 39

Method

1. In a small saucepan, combine green pepper and water. Cover and cook over low heat until tender, about 5 to 7 minutes.
2. Drain any excess liquid.
3. In a blender, combine peppers, pimento, hot pepper sauce, garlic and olive oil; purée until smooth.
4. Stir in bread crumbs.
5. Taste and adjust seasonings with hot pepper sauce.

Pepperonata

2 tbsp.	olive oil	25 mL
2	medium onions, sliced	2
1	clove garlic, minced	1
4	large sweet red, green or yellow peppers, seeded and cut in ½ inch (1 cm) strips	4
1½ cups	chopped tomatoes	375 mL
1 tsp.	red wine vinegar	5 mL
½ tsp.	dried oregano	2 mL
⅛ tsp.	salt	0.5 mL
	freshly ground pepper	

Method

1. In a large non-stick saucepan or skillet, heat oil over medium heat. Add onion and garlic; sauté for 6 to 8 minutes or until golden.
2. Add peppers; sauté for 3 minutes.
3. Reduce heat; cover and simmer for about 15 minutes.
4. Add tomatoes, vinegar, oregano, salt and pepper; cover and simmer for 12 to 15 minutes or until peppers are almost tender.
5. Uncover and increase heat to medium-high; cook until most of the liquid has evaporated, stirring often.
6. Taste and add more pepper if desired.

Sweet and colorful with a variety of peppers, this is a late summer classic accompaniment to grilled meats. Why not try it with turkey in a pita or dress up a plain omelet or serve it on focaccia as an appetizer.

Makes 4 cups (1 L)

1/2 Cup:
Protein 1 gram
Fat 3 grams
Carbohydrate 7 grams
Calories 59

The fastest racquetball serve ever officially clocked was 179 miles per hour.

Raspberry Coulis

Magnificent with fresh straw-berries, this fruity sauce tops ice cream or cheesecake equally well.

Makes about 1 cup (250 mL)

2 Tablespoons:
Carbohydrate 5 grams
Calories 20

1	300 g package frozen unsweetened raspberries, thawed OR 1¼ cups (300 mL) fresh raspberries	1
¼ cup	icing sugar	50 mL

Method
1. In a blender or food processor, purée raspberries.
2. Press through a sieve to remove seeds.
3. Whisk sugar into purée.
4. Serve immediately or cover and refrigerate for up to 3 days.

Vanilla Sauce

Makes a quick dessert when added to fresh fruit and topped with Truly Healthy Granola (page 75).

Makes 1/2 cup (125 mL)

2 Tablespoons:
Protein 1 gram
Carbohydrate 2.5 grams
Calories 14
Fat trace

1	egg white	1
¼ cup	2% plain yogurt	50 mL
2 tsp.	granulated sugar	10 mL
¼ tsp.	vanilla	1 mL

Method
1. Beat egg white until foamy and soft peaks form; fold in yogurt, sugar and vanilla.
2. Serve immediately over warm fruit crisp, baked apples or fresh fruits.
3. Sauce will separate upon standing; beat with a fork to reblend.

Baked Goods and Desserts:
sweet taste of victory

Pear Bread Pudding

½ loaf	day-old egg bread, sliced ¼ inch thick	½ loaf
1 tbsp.	butter	15 mL
5	pears, peeled, cored, and cut into ½ inch wedges	5
½ cup	sugar	125 mL
½ cup	raisins, plumped in hot water or rum	125 mL
2½ cups	1% milk	625 mL
3	eggs	3
1 tsp.	vanilla	5 mL
½ tsp.	cinnamon	2 mL

Tender, slightly caramelized pears give this centuries-old favorite a touch of elegance. Prepared in minutes, this custardy treat can be enjoyed warm from the oven for dessert or as a special breakfast.

Method
1. Preheat oven to 350°F (180°C).
2. Lightly grease 9 inch pie plate, tart pan or baking dish. Cut bread slices into 4 squares; arrange half the bread in single layer in prepared dish.
3. Melt butter in a large skillet over medium heat; add pears and sauté 5 minutes. Sprinkle with 2 tbsp. sugar; cook another 5 minutes, or until pears are golden. Arrange pears over bread. Sprinkle with raisins. Cover with remaining bread.
4. In a small saucepan, bring milk to a simmer. In a large bowl, whisk together eggs and remaining sugar. Whisk in hot milk, vanilla and cinnamon. Pour over bread and pear mixture. Let stand until milk mixture is almost absorbed, about 30 minutes.
5. Place dish in roasting pan. Add enough hot water to come halfway up sides of dish. Bake bread pudding until top is golden and custard is set, about 1 hour. Remove from water. Serve warm or at room temperature.

Serves 4 to 6

1 Serving:
Protein 11 grams
Fat 7 grams
Carbohydrate 74 grams
Calories 403

Frozen Peach Yogurt

A light, low fat, delicious alternative to ice cream, this frosty dessert gets its inspiration from a popular drink, the daiquiri.

2 cups	sliced fresh or frozen unsweetened peaches	500 mL
1 cup	2% plain yogurt	250 mL
¼ cup	granulated sugar	50 mL
1 tbsp.	light rum	15 mL
1 tsp.	lime juice	5 mL
½ tsp.	grated lime rind	2 mL
	mint leaves and/or fresh fruit for garnish	

Makes 4 to 6 servings

1 Serving:
Protein 3 grams
Fat 0.5 gram
Carbohydrate 17 grams
Calories 84

Method

1. In blender or food processor, combine peaches, yogurt, sugar, rum, lime juice and rind; process until smooth.
2. **Freeze** in an ice-cream maker according to manufacturer's directions. OR **pour** into a shallow baking pan and freeze until almost firm; spoon into food processor and process until almost smooth
   or beat with electric mixer. Transfer to freezer container and freeze until firm.
3. To serve, remove from freezer 10 to 15 minutes before serving.
4. To give a creamier texture, process a second time just before serving if desired.
5. Scoop into sherbet dishes or glasses.
6. Garnish with mint leaves or fresh fruit.

Serving Suggestion

Peach Melba: Place a scoop of frozen yogurt in a glass dish. Arrange fresh peach slices around it. Drizzle with 2 tbsp. (25 mL) Raspberry Coulis (page 218). Garnish with mint.

Dumitru Dan of Romania was the only man out of 200 entrants to succeed in walking 62,137 miles, in a contest organized by the Touring Club de France on April 1, 1910. By March 24, 1916, he had covered 59,651 miles, averaging 27.24 miles per day.

Orange Poached Pears

1	pear, ripe but firm	1	
¼ cup	orange juice	50 mL	
1 tbsp.	honey	15 mL	
1 tsp.	lemon juice	5 mL	
½ tsp.	cornstarch	2 mL	
	grated orange rind and/or mint leaves for garnish		

Bosc or Bartlett pears are the best variety for poaching.

Method

1. Halve pear lengthwise; peel and core.
2. Pour orange juice and honey into a 7 inch (17 cm) skillet or saucepan.
3. Place pear halves cut side down in skillet.
4. Bring to boil; reduce heat and simmer for 8 to 10 minutes or until cooked but firm.
5. Remove pears and place each half on serving plate.
6. Mix lemon juice and cornstarch together; add to hot juice in skillet.
7. Cook and stir for 1 to 2 minutes, stirring until thickened and clear.
8. Pour over pears.
9. Serve warm or chilled, garnished with orange rind or mint.

Makes 2 servings

1 Serving:
Protein 1 gram
Fat 1 gram
Carbohydrate 24 grams
Calories 109

Moroccan Oranges

2	seedless navel oranges	2	
¼ cup	dry white wine	50 mL	
2 tsp.	icing sugar	10 mL	
¼ tsp.	ground cinnamon	1 mL	
2 tbsp.	pomegranate seeds for garnish	25 mL	

A warm taste in a cool, refreshing dessert.

Method

1. Using sharp knife, peel oranges, removing pith.
2. Slice oranges ¼ inch (0.5 cm) thick.
3. Arrange slices in 2 serving dishes or plates, overlapping if necessary.
4. Mix wine, sugar and cinnamon together.
5. Spoon over orange slices.
6. Cover and refrigerate for 30 minutes or overnight.
7. Sprinkle pomegranate seeds over top if using.

Makes 2 servings

1 Serving:
Protein 1 gram
Carbohydrate 19 grams
Calories 80

High Energy
Oatmeal Cookies

This is a moist, chewy cookie that is a perfect totable for brown bag or backpack.

¾ cup	brown sugar	175 mL
⅓ cup	butter or soft margarine	75 mL
1 tsp.	vanilla	5 mL
½ cup	whole wheat flour	125 mL
1 tsp.	ground cinnamon	5 mL
½ tsp.	baking soda	2 mL
¼ tsp.	salt	1 mL
1¾ cups	rolled oats	425 mL
½ cup	mini-chocolate chips or raisins	125 mL
¼ cup	water	50 mL

Method

1. In a medium bowl, beat sugar, butter and vanilla together for 3 to 4 minutes or until well mixed and creamy.
2. In a separate bowl, mix flour, cinnamon, soda and salt together.
3. Add to sugar mixture; mix well.
4. Stir in rolled oats, chips and water.
5. Drop by tablespoonfuls about 2 inches (5 cm) apart on a non-stick cookie sheet or on a cookie sheet lined with parchment paper.
6. Bake in 350°F (180°C) oven for 12 to 15 minutes or until golden around the edges.

Makes about 2 dozen cookies

1 Cookie:
Protein 1.5 grams
Fat 4 grams
Carbohydrate 13 grams
Calories 94

Trail Bar

Chewy, crunchy and a natural high-energy bar, this packs easily for a quick pick-me-up deep in the woods or at the office.

¾ cup	corn syrup	175 mL
½ cup	brown sugar, lightly packed	125 mL
1½ cups	chunky peanut butter	375 mL
1 cup	skim milk powder	250 mL
1 cup	Truly Healthy Granola (page 75)	250 mL
1 cup	natural wheat bran	250 mL
1 cup	raisins	250 mL
1 cup	mini-chocolate chips (optional)	250 mL

Method

1. In a large saucepan, combine corn syrup and sugar; bring to boil.
2. Remove from heat; stir in peanut butter until smooth.
3. Stir in milk powder, granola, bran, raisins and chocolate chips if using.
4. Press into 9 x 13 inch (3.5 L) pan.
5. Chill for 45 minutes.
6. Cut into bars and store in refrigerator.

Makes about 3 dozen bars

1 Bar:
Protein 5 grams
Fat 6 grams
Carbohydrate 18 grams
Calories 146

Oat Squares

1½ cups	sliced pitted prunes	375 mL
¾ cup	orange juice	175 mL
2 tsp.	grated orange rind	10 mL
1 cup	rolled oats	250 mL
1 cup	whole wheat flour	250 mL
½ cup	brown sugar	125 mL
¼ cup	oat bran	50 mL
½ tsp.	baking powder	2 mL
½ tsp.	nutmeg	2 mL
½ cup	butter or soft margarine	125 mL
1 tbsp.	water	15 mL

Method

1. In a 1 qt. (1 L) microwaveable measure, combine prunes, orange juice and rind.
2. Cover with plastic wrap and microwave at High for 5 to 6 minutes or until liquid is almost absorbed, stirring once.
3. Let stand covered for 5 minutes.
4. In a large bowl, combine rolled oats, flour, sugar, oat bran, baking powder and nutmeg.
5. With 2 knives, cut in butter until mixture is crumbly.
6. Sprinkle water over mixture; toss to mix well.
7. Press half the mixture into bottom of lightly greased 8 inch (20 cm) square baking pan.
8. Spread with prune filling; top with remaining crumb mixture, patting down firmly.
9. Bake in 350°F (180°C) oven for 25 to 30 minutes or until lightly browned.
10. Cool on rack. Cut into squares.

These citrus-prune bars are addictive. Rich in flavor not to mention nutrients, prunes and oat bran give this sweet snack high fiber.

Makes 25 squares

1 Square:
Protein 2 grams
Fat 4 grams
Carbohydrate 20 grams
Calories 124

Apricot Truffles

A gem of a no-bake treat, the ginger packs a punch in these candies that are a perfect ending to any sports day.

Makes 2 to 3 dozen

1 Truffle:
Fat 0.5 gram
Carbohydrate 5 grams
Calories 24

1 cup	Jane's Apricot Conserve (page 80)	250 mL
⅓ cup	graham wafer crumbs	75 mL
1 to 2 tbsp.	finely diced preserved stem ginger	15 to 25 mL
1 tbsp.	liquid honey	15 mL
½ cup	unsweetened desiccated coconut	125 mL

Method

1. In a medium bowl, combine conserve, crumbs, ginger and honey; mix well.
2. Drop rounded teaspoonfuls into coconut.
3. Toss to coat well and roll into balls.
4. Store in airtight container in a cool place for up to 1 month.

Berry Berry Shortcake

This is a wholesome update on a North American summer favorite.

Makes 4 servings

1 Serving:
Protein 7 grams
Fat 9 grams
Carbohydrate 49 grams
Calories 305

2 cups	fresh fruit (strawberries, raspberries, blueberries, and/or sliced peaches)	500 mL
1 cup	Raspberry Coulis (page 218)	250 mL
4	Whole Wheat Shortcakes (page 226)	4
½ cup	Creamy Cheese Topping (below)	125 mL
	fresh fruit pieces and mint leaves for garnish	

Method

1. In a bowl, gently stir fruit with Raspberry Coulis.
2. Cut biscuits in half horizontally; spread each biscuit bottom with half of the Creamy Cheese Topping.
3. Evenly spoon three-quarters of the fruit mixture over the biscuits letting it run over the sides.
4. Replace tops of biscuits; spoon remaining fruit sauce on top.
5. Top each biscuit with a dollop of cheese topping and garnish with fresh fruit and mint.

Creamy Cheese Topping: In a blender or food processor, purée ¼ cup (50 mL) 2% cottage cheese and ¼ cup (50 mL) light cream cheese until smooth. Stir in 1 tbsp. (15 mL) icing sugar and 1 tsp. (5 mL) grated orange rind.

Grapefruit Alaska

1	grapefruit, halved	1	
1 tbsp.	orange liqueur or orange juice	15 mL	
1	egg white	1	
1 tbsp.	sugar	15 mL	
¼ cup	Jane's Apricot Conserve (page 80)	50 mL	
	OR low calorie apricot jam		

This is a cozy dessert perfect after an intimate dinner for two. Toasted golden meringue tops the liqueur-laced grapefruit worthy of an Olympic medal.

Method

1. Remove core of grapefruit with kitchen shears or grapefruit knife; remove seeds.
2. Loosen sections of grapefruit with grapefruit knife, cutting between the flesh and pith and skin so flesh is completely detached from the shell.
3. Spoon liqueur or juice over grapefruit.
4. Beat egg white until soft peaks form; gradually add sugar, beating until stiff peaks form and mixture is glossy.
5. Fold apricot conserve into beaten egg white fold. (If using purchased apricot jam, warm slightly to soften.)
6. Spread over grapefruit halves.
7. Bake in 400°F (200°C) oven for 7 to 9 minutes or until browned.
8. Serve immediately.

Variation

Broiled Grapefruit: Prepare grapefruit as directed in recipe. Mix ¼ cup (50 mL) Jane's Apricot Conserve (page 80), 2 tbsp. (25 mL) orange liqueur or orange juice and 1 tbsp. (15 mL) honey together. Spread over grapefruit halves; broil 4 inches (10 cm) from heat for 4 to 5 minutes or until browned and bubbling. Great for brunch or dessert.

Makes 2 servings

1 Serving:
Protein 1.5 grams
Carbohydrate 30 grams
Calories 126

Whole Wheat Shortcake

Tasty and wholesome with berries for dessert or a nice change from toast for breakfast, these biscuits are tender and wheaty.

¾ cup	buttermilk or sour milk	175 mL
½ cup	natural wheat bran	125 mL
¾ cup	whole wheat flour	175 mL
½ cup	all-purpose flour	125 mL
1 tbsp.	granulated sugar	15 mL
1 tsp.	baking powder	5 mL
1 tsp.	grated lemon rind	5 mL
1 tsp.	grated orange rind	5 mL
½ tsp.	baking soda	2 mL
⅛ tsp.	salt	0.5 mL
¼ cup	butter or soft margarine	0.5 mL

Method

1. In a small bowl, combine buttermilk and bran; set aside.
2. In a medium bowl, combine whole wheat flour, all-purpose flour, sugar, baking powder, lemon and orange rind, baking soda and salt.
3. Cut in butter with 2 knives until coarse crumbs are formed.
4. Add reserved bran mixture. Stir to mix well with a fork.
5. Turn out onto lightly floured surface. Pat or roll dough to ¾ inch (1.5 cm) thickness.
6. Using a 2½ inch (6 cm) cookie cutter, cut out rounds.
7. Press and knead scraps of dough together and repeat.
8. Place rounds on non-stick baking sheet. Bake in 400°F (200°C) oven for 15 to 20 minutes or until lightly browned.
9. Serve warm.

Makes 6 shortcakes

1 Biscuit:
Protein 4 grams
Fat 7 grams
Carbohydrate 25 grams
Calories 179

Tip
To sour milk, use 1 tbsp. (15 mL) lemon juice and add 2% milk to make 3/4 cup (175 mL).

Honey Cheesecake

Crust:

1	3.5 oz (100 g) package whole wheat rusks or zwieback	1
½ to 1 tsp.	ground cinnamon	2 to 5 mL
¼ cup	butter or soft margarine, melted	50 mL
2 tbsp.	honey	25 mL
1 tbsp.	water	15 mL

Filling:

1½ cups	ricotta cheese (about 12 oz/375 g)	375 mL
2	eggs, separated	2
⅓ cup	honey	75 mL
1 tbsp.	cornstarch	15 mL
½ cup	canned 2% evaporated milk	125 mL
1 tbsp.	lemon juice	15 mL
1 tbsp.	grated lemon rind	15 mL
1 tsp.	vanilla	5 mL
1	egg white	1
	Raspberry Coulis (page 218) for garnish	

Distinctively sweet from the honey, this creamy rich European-style cheesecake is superb served on Raspberry Coulis.

Method

1. Break rusks into food processor bowl; process to crush to fine crumbs.
2. In an 8 inch (20 cm) springform pan or in an 8 inch (20 cm) square baking pan, mix crumbs and cinnamon.
3. In a small measure, mix butter, honey and water; add to crumbs.
4. Mix well and press onto bottom and about 1 inch (2.5 cm) up sides of pan.
5. Bake in 325°F (160°C) oven for 7 to 8 minutes.
6. In blender or food processor bowl, combine cheese, egg yolks, honey and cornstarch. Process until smooth.
7. Add milk, lemon juice, rind and vanilla; process until well blended.
8. In a large bowl, beat the 3 egg whites until soft peaks form; fold cheese mixture into egg whites. Pour into crust.
9. Bake in 325°F (160°C) oven for 35 to 40 minutes or just until set (it may still quiver in the middle).
10. Remove and cool on rack 10 minutes; loosen around edge with a straight knife. Cool completely for about 40 to 50 minutes.
11. Cover with plastic wrap and chill for 6 hours or overnight.
12. Cut into wedges or squares and serve each piece on a pool of Raspberry Coulis.

Makes 8 servings

1 Serving:
Protein 10 grams
Fat 13 grams
Carbohydrate 27 grams
Calories 265

Chocolate Pudding

Creamy, chocolaty, easy and low fat...what more could you ask for?

2 tbsp.	cornstarch	25 mL
¼ cup	cocoa powder	50 mL
½ cup	sugar	125 mL
2	large egg yolks	2
1 tsp.	almond extract (optional)	5 mL
1 tsp.	vanilla	5 mL
¼ tsp.	salt	1 mL
2 cups	1% milk	500 mL

Makes 2 cups
Serves 4 to 6

1 Serving:
Protein 5 grams
Fat 4 grams
Carbohydrate 26 grams
Calories 160

Method

1. In a medium bowl, combine the cornstarch and cocoa powder. In a separate bowl, whisk together the sugar, yolks, almond extract (if using), vanilla and salt.
2. Place the milk in a large saucepan, and over medium heat, bring just to a boil; remove from heat and whisk a small amount into the cornstarch mixture.
3. Return to saucepan, heat, and cook, stirring constantly, until milk begins to bubble around the edges. Simmer gently, stirring, for about 2 minutes. Remove from heat.
4. Whisk 1 cup of hot liquid into yolk mixture and scrape back into saucepan. Cook over medium heat, stirring constantly, until thickened, about 3 minutes.
5. Pour into serving dish or divide among ramekins. Chill for several hours before serving. May be refrigerated for up to 1 day.

Kiwi Sorbet

For a pretty presentation, alternate scoops of Kiwi Sorbet and Frozen Peach Yogurt with seasonal fruits.

6	kiwis, peeled and quartered	6
⅓ cup	granulated sugar	75 mL
4 tsp.	lemon juice	20 mL
1	egg white	1

Makes 4 servings

1 Serving:
Protein 1 gram
Carbohydrate 38 grams
Calories 156

Method

1. In a blender or food processor, combine kiwi, sugar, lemon juice and egg white; blend just until smooth. (Don't over-process or kiwi seeds will be crushed, creating a bitterness.)
2. Freeze in ice-cream maker or as directed in Frozen Peach Yogurt recipe (page 220).

Raspberry Yogurt Mousse

1	7 g envelope unflavored gelatine	1
¼ cup	cold water	50 mL
1	425 g package frozen raspberries in light syrup, thawed	1
1 cup	2% plain yogurt	250 mL
3 tbsp.	icing sugar	50 mL
1 tbsp	lemon juice	15 mL
2	egg whites	2
2 tbsp.	granulated sugar	25 mL
	fresh or frozen and thawed whole raspberries for garnish	
	lemon zest for garnish	

Tart and refreshing, this creamy light dessert is a fitting close to a meal of celebration.

Method

1. In a small saucepan, sprinkle gelatine over cold water and allow to soften for 3 to 4 minutes; heat over low heat, stirring constantly until dissolved. Set aside to cool.
2. In a blender or food processor, purée raspberries with syrup; strain purée into a large bowl to remove seeds.
3. Beat in yogurt, icing sugar and lemon juice with a fork or whisk; stir in gelatine mixture.
4. In a small bowl, beat egg whites until soft peaks form; gradually add sugar while continuing to beat until stiff peaks form.
5. Fold egg whites into raspberry yogurt mixture.
6. Pour into a 4 cup (1 L) soufflé dish, glass bowl or 8 wine or sherbet glasses.
7. Cover and refrigerate until set, at least one hour or overnight.
8. Garnish with raspberries or lemon zest.

Makes 8 servings

1 Serving:
Protein 3 grams
Fat 0.5 gram
Carbohydrate 20 grams
Calories 96

The first recognizable swimming stroke style seems to have been the breaststroke, although the "dog paddle" technique may well have preceded it.

Sesame Corn Bread

A new twist on the southern classic, this quick bread is the consummate companion to chili, soups, cheese spreads.

1 cup	all-purpose flour	250 mL
1 cup	yellow cornmeal	250 mL
⅓ cup	wheat germ	75 mL
¼ cup	toasted sesame seeds or chopped pumpkin or sunflower seeds	50 mL
2 tbsp.	granulated sugar	25 mL
1 tbsp.	baking powder	15 mL
¼ tsp.	salt	1 mL
1 cup	2% milk	250 mL
2	eggs	2
⅓ cup	vegetable oil	75 mL

Makes 16 squares

1 Square:

Protein 4 grams

Fat 6 grams

Carbohydrate 17 grams

Calories 138

Method

1. In a medium bowl, combine flour, cornmeal, wheat germ, sesame seeds, sugar, baking powder and salt.
2. In a large bowl, mix milk, eggs and oil together; add dry ingredients and stir just until moistened.
3. Pour into 8 inch (2 L) square non-stick pan.
4. Bake in 375°F (190°C) for 25 to 30 minutes or until golden brown.
5. Cut in squares.

Variation

Southwestern Style: Add 1 can (4 oz/114 mL) diced drained green chilies or jalapeno peppers to the mixture. Bake as in recipe.

Dried Fruit Compote with Yogurt Cheese

2 cups	plain non-fat yogurt	500 mL
1 cup	water	250 mL
½ cup	Cointreau or Triple Sec	125 mL
½ cup	brown sugar	125 mL
2 tbsp.	lemon juice	25 mL
3	orange-spice teabags	3
½ cup	dried apricots	125 mL
½ cup	pitted prunes	125 mL
½ cup	dried cranberries	125 mL

Method

1. *Yogurt Cheese:* Set strainer over medium bowl. Line strainer with double layer of cheesecloth. Place yogurt in strainer. Refrigerate overnight, or until reduced by a third. Discard liquid that drains out.
2. Combine water, Cointreau, brown sugar and lemon juice, in small saucepan. Bring to a boil, stirring until sugar dissolves. Add teabags, submerging them completely. Add fruit and simmer about 5 minutes, or until liquid is syrupy and fruit is plumped. Remove from heat; remove teabags and cool.
3. Cover and refrigerate for at least 1 hour or until completely chilled.
4. Place heaping spoonful of yogurt cheese in center of each bowl. Surround with fruit compote. Drizzle with any remaining syrup.

Variations:

In warmer weather, try seasonal fruits as accompaniments to the yogurt cheese.
Using the same method, combine strawberries, bananas, kiwis and melons with mint tea; or, combine citrus fruits such as oranges and grapefruits with Grand Marnier.

Dried fruit is intensely flavored as well as packed with nutrients and fiber. This comforting fruit mélange partners perfectly with spiced tea, a hint of liqueur and the thick, creamy yogurt topping.

Serves 4

1 Serving:
Protein 7 grams
Fat 3 grams
Carbohydrate 75 grams
Calories 355

Fresh Fruit Brûlé

Sophisticated version of a warm, citrusy custard.

1 tbsp.	granulated sugar	15 mL
1 tsp.	cornstarch	5 mL
1	egg	1
½ cup	2% milk	125 mL
1 tbsp.	orange liqueur	15 mL
½ tsp.	grated orange rind	2 mL
1 cup	fresh blueberries, raspberries or strawberries	250 mL
1 tsp.	brown sugar	5 mL

Makes 2 servings

1 Serving:
Protein 6 grams
Fat 4 grams
Carbohydrate 20 grams
Calories 140

Method

1. In a small saucepan, combine sugar and cornstarch.
2. Beat egg and milk together, gradually stir into sugar mixture.
3. Cook over low heat, stirring or whisking constantly until thickened.
4. Remove from heat; cool for 5 minutes.
5. Stir in liqueur and orange rind.
6. Cover surface with plastic wrap and chill until serving time.
7. At serving time, divide fruit among 2 oven-proof ramekins.
8. Spoon custard mixture over fruit. Sprinkle with brown sugar.
9. Broil 4 to 5 inches (10 to 13 cm) from heat for 3 to 4 minutes or until sugar caramelizes.

Cranapple Streusel Pie

Crust:

⅔ cup	rolled oats	150 mL
¾ cup	all-purpose flour	175 mL
¼ tsp.	salt	1 mL
¼ cup	butter or cold, soft margarine	50 mL
3 to 4 tbsp.	ice water	45 to 50 mL

Filling:

1 cup	fresh or frozen cranberries	250 mL
¾ cup	frozen unsweetened apple juice concentrate, thawed	175 mL
3 tbsp.	granulated sugar	50 mL
2 tbsp.	cornstarch	25 mL
1 tbsp.	butter or soft margarine	15 mL
1 tsp.	ground cinnamon	5 mL
1 tsp.	vanilla	5 mL
4	apples, peeled, cored and thinly sliced (about 4 cups/1 L)	4
¾ cup	Streusel Topping (page 236)	175 mL

Lots of eye and appetite appeal with this modern version of Mom's favorite. Rich ruby color and vibrant taste are blessed with the wholesome bonus of oats. Top with Vanilla Sauce (page 218) for the ultimate slice.

Method

Crust:

1. In blender or food processor, process rolled oats until finely ground.
2. In a medium bowl, combine ground oats, flour and salt.
3. Cut in butter until mixture resembles coarse meal.
4. Add ice water gradually, tossing after each addition with a fork, until mixture is moist enough to start to cling together.
5. Put mixture into a 9 inch (22 cm) pie plate.
6. Press the mixture onto the bottom and up sides of pie plate allowing it to extend a little above the rim.
7. Flute or crimp the edge with fingers or fork.
8. Cover and chill while preparing filling.

Filling:

1. In a medium saucepan, combine cranberries, apple juice concentrate, sugar and cornstarch.
2. Bring to boil and cook, stirring constantly until mixture has thickened and cranberries have softened, about 5 to 8 minutes.
3. Stir in butter, cinnamon and vanilla; add apples and toss to coat; let cool.
4. Pour into prepared crust.
5. Sprinkle streusel topping over pie.
6. Bake in 425°F (220°C) oven for 15 to 20 minutes or until crust and topping are browned; cover with foil and bake for about 5 minutes longer or until apples are tender.
7. Remove and cool on wire rack.
8. Serve at room temperature.

Makes 6 to 8 servings

1 Serving:
Protein 3.5 grams
Fat 11 grams
Carbohydrate 52 grams
Calories 321

Lemon "Flapper" Pie

Lemon and ginger
complement each other
nicely in this light creamy
finish to a hearty meal.

Crust:

2 tbsp.	butter or soft margarine	25 mL
1 tbsp.	water	15 mL
1¼ cups	gingersnap or ginger cookie crumbs	300 mL

Filling:

¾ cup	granulated sugar, divided	175 mL
⅓ cup	fresh lemon juice	75 mL
¼ cup	cornstarch	50 mL
1 tbsp.	grated lemon rind	15 mL
¾ cup	water	175 mL
1	egg yolk, beaten	1
½ cup	canned evaporated skim milk, well chilled	125 mL
1 tsp.	fresh lemon juice	5 mL
	lemon zest for garnish	
	mint leaves for garnish	

Method

1. Place small mixing bowl, beaters and evaporated milk in freezer to chill well.

Crust:

1. In a 9 inch (22 cm) Pyrex pie plate, microwave butter at High for 40 to 60 seconds or until melted; stir in water.
2. Add crumbs and mix well and press onto bottom and sides of pie plate.
3. **Microwave** at High for 1½ minutes. OR **bake** in 350°F (180°C) oven for 8 to 9 minutes or until set. Let cool.

Filling:

1. In a small saucepan, combine ½ cup (125 mL) of the sugar, lemon juice, cornstarch and rind.
2. With a fork, beat water and egg yolk together; stir into starch mixture.
3. **Cook** over medium-high heat, stirring constantly until thickened. OR **combine** ingredients in 4 cup (1 L) Pyrex measure and microwave at High for 3 to 4 minutes or until thickened,
   stirring twice during cooking.
4. Place in a large bowl and cover surface of filling with plastic wrap; chill for 20 to 30 minutes.
5. In chilled mixing bowl, combine evaporated milk, remaining sugar and 1 tsp. (5 mL) lemon juice.
6. Using chilled beaters, beat on high speed until stiff peaks form.
7. Beat lemon filling with a whisk; fold in half the whipped milk; repeat with remaining whipped milk.
8. Pour into prepared crust and chill for 2 to 3 hours or until set.
9. Garnish with lemon zest and mint leaves.

Makes 6 servings

1 Serving:
Protein 2.5 grams
Fat 4 grams
Carbohydrate 36 grams
Calories 190

Nutty Pumpkin Loaf

1 cup	whole wheat flour	250 mL
½ cup	all-purpose flour	125 mL
½ cup	brown sugar	125 mL
¼ cup	wheat germ	50 mL
2 tsp.	baking powder	10 mL
½ tsp.	ground cinnamon	2 mL
¼ tsp.	baking soda	1 mL
¼ tsp.	salt	1 mL
¼ tsp.	ground allspice	1 mL
¼ tsp.	ground ginger	1 mL
¼ tsp.	ground cloves	1 mL
1 cup	cooked mashed or canned pumpkin	250 mL
½ cup	2% milk	125 mL
⅓ cup	vegetable oil	75 mL
1	egg	1
½ cup	chopped dates	125 mL
½ cup	chopped walnuts	125 mL

The natural sweetness from the dates and pumpkin make this a toothsome treat at home or on the trail.

Method

1. In a medium bowl, combine whole wheat flour, all-purpose flour, sugar, wheat germ, baking powder, cinnamon, baking soda, salt, allspice, ginger and cloves.
2. In a large bowl, beat pumpkin, milk, oil and egg together; add dry ingredients.
3. Mix just until moistened.
4. Fold in dates and nuts and pour into 8½ x 4½ inch (1.5 L) lightly greased loaf pan.
5. Bake in 350°F (180°C) oven for 40 to 45 minutes or until toothpick inserted in center comes out clean.
6. Cool for 10 minutes in pan on rack; remove from pan and cool completely on rack.

Variation

Pumpkin Muffins: Spoon batter into 12 prepared muffin cups. Bake in 350°F (180°C) oven for 15 to 20 minutes or until tops are golden brown and just firm to the touch.

Makes 1 loaf

1 Slice:
Protein 3 grams
Fat 7 grams
Carbohydrate 23 grams
Calories 167

Tip

1 cup (250 mL) cooked pumpkin is about 1/2 can (14 oz./398 mL) so it's easy to double recipe and make 2 loaves – freeze one for later or give one to a friend.

Fruit Crisp

Spring, summer, fall or winter, we love the warm goodness of fruit crisp.

3 cups	thinly sliced apples and/or pears (about 2 medium apples or 2 pears), unpeeled	750 mL
⅓ cup	raisins	75 mL
1 tbsp.	lemon juice	15 mL
1 tbsp.	granulated sugar	15 mL
¾ cup	Streusel Topping (below)	175 mL
	Vanilla Sauce (page 218)	

STREUSEL TOPPING:

¼ cup	whole wheat flour	50 mL
¼ cup	rolled oats	50 mL
¼ cup	oat bran	50 mL
¼ cup	brown sugar	50 mL
2 tsp.	cinnamon	10 mL
¼ cup	butter or soft margarine	50 mL

Makes 4 servings

1 Serving (without sauce):
Protein 3 grams
Fat 10 grams
Carbohydrate 60 grams
Calories 342

Makes about 3/4 cup (175 mL)

Method

1. In an 8 inch (2 L) square, non-stick baking dish or casserole, combine sliced fruit and raisins.
2. Mix lemon juice and sugar with fruit.
3. Sprinkle streusel topping evenly over fruit.
4. Bake in 350°F (180°C) oven for 25 to 30 minutes (depending how thinly fruit is sliced).
5. Serve warm with or without Vanilla Sauce.

Topping:

1. In a small bowl, combine flour, oats, oat bran, sugar and cinnamon.
2. Mix butter in with a fork until crumbly.

Fruit Variations

Blueberry-Apple or Raspberry-Apple: Substitute 1 cup (250 mL) blueberries or raspberries for 1 cup (250 mL) apples in recipe and omit raisins.

Peach-Blueberry: Substitute 2 cups (500 mL) sliced peaches and 1 cup (250 mL) blueberries for 3 cups (750 mL) apples in recipe and omit raisins.

Rhubarb-Strawberry: Substitute 1½ cups (375 mL) strawberries and 1½ cups (375 mL) chopped rhubarb for 3 cups (750 mL) apples in recipe and omit lemon juice and raisins.

Almond Brownie Bites

⅓ cup	butter or soft margarine	75 mL
½ cup	granulated sugar	125 mL
¼ cup	corn syrup	50 mL
1	egg	1
1	egg white	1
⅓ cup	unsweetened cocoa powder	75 mL
¼ cup	all purpose flour	50 mL
¼ cup	oat bran	50 mL
½ tsp.	baking powder	2 mL
¼ tsp.	salt	1 mL
⅓ cup	chopped almonds	75 mL

Chocoholics rejoice – this moist chewy square is densely chocolate without being overly sweet or too high in fat.

Method

1. In a large bowl, beat butter until smooth.
2. Gradually beat in sugar until creamy.
3. Add corn syrup, egg and egg white; beat until well mixed.
4. In a separate bowl, mix cocoa, flour, oat bran, baking powder and salt together; stir into wet ingredients.
5. Stir in nuts.
6. Pour into lightly greased 8 inch (2 L) square pan.
7. Bake in 350°F (180°C) oven for 20 to 25 minutes, or just until toothpick inserted in center comes out clean. Don't overbake.
8. Cool on wire rack.
9. Cut into small squares.

Makes 25 pieces

1 Piece:
Protein 1 gram
Fat 4 grams
Carbohydrate 8 grams
Calories 72

Apple Spice Cake

This spicy, carrot-apple cake is moist, delectable and wholesome.

¼ cup	boiling water	50 mL
½ cup	raisins	125 mL
½ cup	unsweetened applesauce	125 mL
⅓ cup	brown sugar	75 mL
¼ cup	vegetable oil	50 mL
1	egg	1
½ cup	all-purpose flour	125 mL
½ cup	whole wheat flour	125 mL
1 tsp.	baking soda	5 mL
½ tsp.	ground cinnamon	2 mL
½ tsp.	ground nutmeg	2 mL
½ tsp.	ground cloves	2 mL
⅛ tsp.	salt	0.5 mL
½ cup	chopped walnuts	125 mL
½ cup	grated carrot	125 mL
	icing sugar or Creamy Cheese Topping (page 224)	

Makes 12 to 16 slices

1 Slice:
Protein 2 grams
Fat 5 grams
Carbohydrate 15 grams
Calories 113

Method

1. In a small bowl, pour water over raisins; set aside.
2. In a medium bowl, combine applesauce, sugar, oil and egg; mix well.
3. In a separate bowl, stir together all-purpose flour, whole wheat flour, baking soda, cinnamon, nutmeg, cloves and salt.
4. Stir into applesauce mixture until well blended.
5. Stir in walnuts, carrot and raisins with liquid.
6. Pour batter into an 8 inch (2 L) square, non-stick or lightly greased baking pan.
7. Bake in 325°F (160°C) oven for 25 to 30 minutes or until top springs back lightly when touched.
8. Cool on wire rack.
9. Sift icing sugar over top or spread with Creamy Cheese Topping.

Index

About the Authors

Frances Berkoff is a consulting dietitian in Toronto, columnist for the *Toronto Sun* newspaper and outpatient dietitian at Mount Sinai Hospital. Her practice has included athletes, both professional and amateur, as well as sports teams.

Barbara Lauer, a former journalist, is a marketing communications professional who has specialized in food and nutrition for the past 20 years. She's a former columnist for *Images*, *HealthWatch* and *FOOD* magazines.

Dr. Yves Talbot, an internationally respected specialist in Family Medicine, is an Associate Professor of Family Medicine at the University of Toronto. He is the former Chief of Family Medicine at Mount Sinai Hospital in Toronto Ontario, Canada.